THE R.E.P.A.I.R GUIDE TO REVERSING NEUROPATHY

Dr. Jill Althoff, D.C.
The R.E.P.A.I.R Guide to Reversing Neuropathy

Published by Spines
ISBN: 979-8-89691-074-9

THE R.E.P.A.I.R GUIDE TO REVERSING NEUROPATHY

RECLAIM YOUR HEALTH THROUGH NATURAL HEALING

DR. JILL ALTHOFF, D.C.

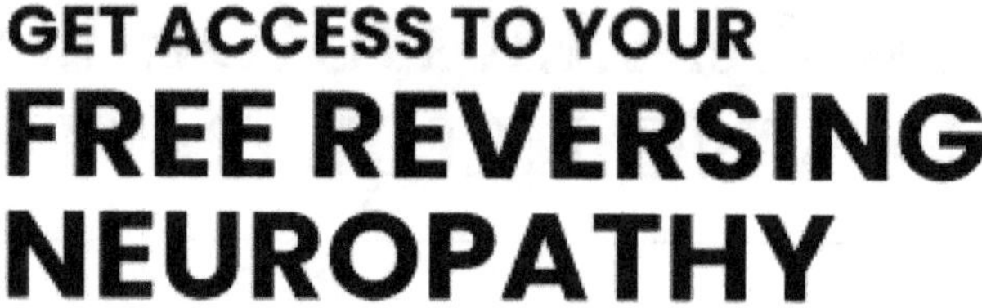

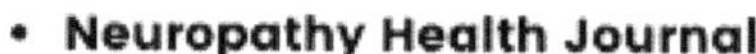

- Neuropathy Health Journal
- Reversing Neuropathy Guide
- 25 Anti-Inflammatory Recipes
- Nerve Damage Quiz
- Free Health Masterclass
- 30-Day Nutrition Plan
- Neuropathy Relief Handbook

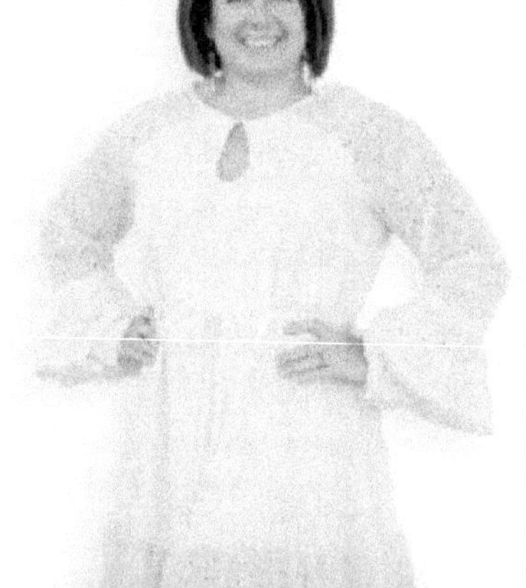

CONTENTS

FOREWORD

In the world of healthcare, it's all too common to hear stories of individuals struggling with the relentless pain, numbness, and tingling sensations of neuropathy. Often, they're told to simply manage their symptoms, leaving them feeling hopeless. But there is reason for hope! There are natural pathways to significantly reduce pain, improve quality of life, and regain control over your health. That path is outlined within the pages of this groundbreaking book, "The R.E.P.A.I.R Guide to Reversing Neuropathy - Reclaim Your Health through Natural Healing" by Dr. Jill Althoff, D.C..

Dr. Althoff, a visionary in the field of chiropractic care and a passionate advocate for those suffering from neuropathy, has dedicated her career to finding real solutions for this often-misunderstood condition.

Through her tireless research, clinical experience, and unwavering commitment to her patients, she has developed the R.E.P.A.I.R. Neuropathy Program, a comprehensive and evidence-based approach that is truly changing lives.

As a fellow practitioner and a member of the esteemed Driven Doc community at The Data Driven Practice, I have had the privilege of witnessing firsthand the transformative power of Dr. Althoff's work. Her passion, expertise, and unwavering belief in her patients' ability to heal are nothing short of inspiring.

Through this book, Dr. Althoff generously shares her knowledge and experience, demystifying the complexities of neuropathy and providing a clear roadmap for recovery. The R.E.P.A.I.R. Neuropathy Program is not simply a treatment plan; it is a beacon of hope, a testament to the resilience of the human spirit, and a guide toward reclaiming a life filled with vitality and joy.

With Dr. Althoff and her dedicated team at Althoff Wellness Clinic PC, a leading chiropractic clinic in Windsor, Colorado and Cheyenne, Wyoming by your side, you are not alone on this journey. This book is your first step toward understanding and overcoming neuropathy. Embrace the information within these pages, and I have no doubt that you will find the strength, courage, and knowledge to transform your health and well-being.

Sincerely,

Dr. Cory Frogley, D.C.
The Data Driven Practice

DISCLAIMER

The information provided in this book is intended for educational purposes only and is not a substitute for professional medical advice. The author and publisher are not liable for any adverse effects or consequences resulting from the use of the information presented herein. Always consult your physician or a qualified healthcare provider regarding any health concerns or before making any decisions related to your health or treatment.

Results may vary depending on individual conditions and adherence to the recommended care plan. No claims are made regarding the guaranteed reversal or cure of neuropathy or any other conditions. Testimonials reflect individual patient experiences and are not a promise of specific results. The consultation and any treatments discussed are intended to evaluate your condition and explore potential benefits, but no specific outcomes are guaranteed. This advertisement is not a substitute for professional medical advice. Please consult Dr. Jill Althoff, D.C., for a personalized assessment of your health condition.

ABOUT THE AUTHOR

Since 2003, Dr. Jill Althoff, D.C., has been dedicated to helping people live healthier lives and regain normal function through a holistic approach encompassing six essential pillars of health: spiritual and mental well-being, optimal nervous system function, balanced nutrition, regular exercise, adequate rest, and the elimination of toxins and chemical stressors.

Dr. Althoff's journey into healthcare was profoundly influenced by her personal struggles with asthma and injuries from gymnastics and a motor vehicle accident. Despite being under the care of top specialists, her asthma continued to worsen until she discovered chiropractic care. This natural approach not only alleviated her spine-related issues but also significantly improved her asthma, igniting her passion for holistic health care.

She began her career with a focus on typical chiropractic treatments for back and neck pain, headaches, and nerve pain. However, her drive to help those who didn't respond to conventional treatments led her to specialize in neuropathy. Witnessing the struggles of a patient with severe neuropathy, she was determined to find a better solution than just masking symptoms with medication. This quest led her to extensive research, training, and collaboration with other doctors.

Dr. Althoff developed the REPAIR Neuropathy Program, which stands for Root Cause Discovery, Eliminate Contributing Factors, Pain Relief, Activate Healing, Improve Lifestyle, and Retain Results. This program is designed to help patients reverse nerve damage, reduce pain, improve balance, and regain their quality of life.

Over the years, Dr. Althoff has helped thousands of patients achieve a better quality of life through her holistic approach and the REPAIR Neuropathy Program. Her dedication to continuous improvement and patient care has earned her recognition as one of the top professionals in her field. She currently practices in Windsor, Colorado, and Cheyenne, Wyoming, where she enjoys seeing her patients regain their independence and vitality.

Dr. Althoff holds a Bachelor of Science in Human Biology and a Doctor of Chiropractic degree from North Dakota State College of Science and

Northwestern Health Sciences University. She is board-certified in neuropathy and holds additional certifications in pediatrics, Trigenix, and acupuncture. She lives near Pierce, Colorado, with her husband Josh and their two children, Colten and Caiden. When not helping patients, she enjoys camping, boating, riding ATVs, and playing sports with her family.

In "The R.E.P.A.I.R Guide to Reversing Neuropathy," Dr. Althoff shares her extensive knowledge and experience to help readers achieve the same success and happiness she has seen in her patients.

1

WHO'S TO BLAME FOR AMERICA'S HEALTH CRISIS?

When considering the health crisis in the United States, the discussion often centers around health insurance. Many point fingers at various entities for the current state of affairs:

- **Government:** Blamed for the lack of universal and affordable health insurance.
- **Pharmaceutical Companies:** Criticized for the escalating prices of prescription drugs.
- **Healthcare Industry:** Accused of poor management and inefficient practices.
- **Food Industry:** Held responsible for promoting cheap, highly processed, and unhealthy foods, especially to lower-income individuals.

While each of these parties plays a role in perpetuating the crisis, none of them is the sole cause. The root problem lies in individual choices and lifestyles, particularly in areas of diet, exercise, and stress management. These choices lead to a range of health issues, including cancer, heart disease, metabolic syndrome, stroke, diabetes, and more. Like it or not, personal responsibility for health is crucial. This means educating ourselves about the choices that can make a positive change for us and our loved ones.

The Obesity Epidemic

One of the most pressing health issues in the United States is obesity. It's an epidemic. Among Americans aged 20 and over, 154.7 million are overweight or obese. According to the National Health and Nutrition Examination Survey (NHANES) from 2017–2020, 41.9% of adults in the United States aged 20 and older were obese, up from 30.5% in 1999–2000. A 2023 study published in Population Studies linked obesity and excess weight to around 1 in 6 deaths in the United States, primarily from type 2 diabetes, hypertension, heart disease, liver disease, cancer, dementia, and depression.

The Evolution of the American Diet

How did the obesity problem get so big? Early in the 20th century, the American diet was vastly different. If you could hop in a time machine and peek at the local store your grandparents shopped at, you would find fresh produce, living plants, seeds, and grains. You might also find some home-canned products. You wouldn't find today's grocery store travesties like hormone-injected meats, processed foods, fast foods, and junk foods. With these "modern" choices comes a completely different diet – the Standard American Diet (SAD).

The Impact of Government Intervention

In the mid-20th century, the government became concerned about the amount of salt in the American diet, linking high salt intake to health issues like hypertension. A massive public health campaign was launched to reduce salt consumption. Food manufacturers responded by removing salt from their products. However, they quickly discovered that salt wasn't just a preservative – it was a key flavor enhancer. To compensate for the bland taste of low-salt foods, they began adding sugar. Lots of sugar. As a result, while Americans' salt intake decreased, their sugar consumption skyrocketed. This shift contributed to the rise of obesity, diabetes, and other metabolic diseases.

The Standard American Diet (SAD)

The SAD diet is out of balance in many ways:

- High in Meats, Fats, and Sugar: Overconsumption of animal products and added sugars.
- Low in Fruits and Vegetables: Insufficient intake of nutrient-rich produce.
- Lacking in Nutrients: Overcooking and processing strips foods of their natural benefits.

The Cost of Processed Foods

Companies work tirelessly to make perfect foods like fruits, vegetables, and grains "better" by refining, processing, and adding chemicals to them. This tinkering has created an American diet deficient in many ways. Processed foods make up a huge percentage of the American diet, loaded with extra salt, sugar, artificial flavors, preservatives, and other chemicals. These foods also lack vital nutrients and vitamins that are stripped away during processing. This adding and subtracting from our food is a recipe for disaster. Whole, natural foods are perfect as they are, providing a wide variety of fruits, vegetables, and grains will give your body everything it needs for good health.

The True Health Crisis

The Standard American Diet is high in calories and low in nutrition. To be healthy, we need to replace low-nutrient foods with high-nutrient, non-processed foods, including vegetables, fruits, lean meats in moderation, and fish. A healthy body needs a diet high in vitamins, minerals, enzymes, and antioxidants to ensure proper digestion, nutrient absorption, cell function regulation, and to keep the body fueled up. When your body lacks the nutrients it needs, the aging process speeds up, leading to diseases associated with aging, such as coronary heart disease, stroke, high blood pressure, cancer, diabetes, and osteoporosis.

The Healthcare System: Spending vs. Outcome

The U.S. healthcare system often faces criticism for inefficiencies and high costs. In 2022, U.S. healthcare spending grew by 4.1 percent, reaching $4.5 trillion or $13,493 per person. Despite spending the most on healthcare worldwide, Americans visit doctors less frequently than those in other high-income countries. The World Health Organization (WHO) ranked the United States 37th out of 191 countries in 2000 for its health system performance. In 2021, the Commonwealth Fund ranked the U.S. last overall among high-income countries due to poor performance in areas such as access to care, administrative efficiency, equity, and health outcomes.

Prevention Over Cure

The real answer to the healthcare crisis lies not in modern medicine alone but in the prevention of disease through a healthy lifestyle. Understanding what constitutes a healthy lifestyle can be daunting for many people. However, living healthily involves simple, practical steps:

- **Eat Well:** Eliminate the SAD diet and replace it with fresh fruits and vegetables, whole grains, lean meats, healthy fats, and fish.
- **Exercise Regularly:** Just 30 minutes of exercise three times a week promotes heart health, helps with weight loss, increases metabolism, builds strong bones, and boosts the immune system.
- **Sleep Well:** Adequate sleep is crucial for memory assimilation and repair. Most people need seven to eight hours of sleep each night to function at their best.

- **Live Well:** Embrace kindness, love, and a set of principles to guide your life. This will help you be healthier and live longer.
- **Maintain Nervous System Health:** Everything that happens in our body begins with the nervous system. Removing blockages in the nervous system, known as subluxations, can help you reach your full potential.

Personal Responsibility

The burden of achieving good health falls squarely on your shoulders. You cannot rely on others to watch out for your health. You won't find good health in a doctor's office or in the pharmacy. It's not in the junk food aisles of the grocery store or in fast food restaurants. Health can only be found when you commit to a healthy lifestyle. By taking care of your body now, learning everything you can to make good choices, and finding practitioners that promote the prevention of disease, you will be well on your way to a healthier you.

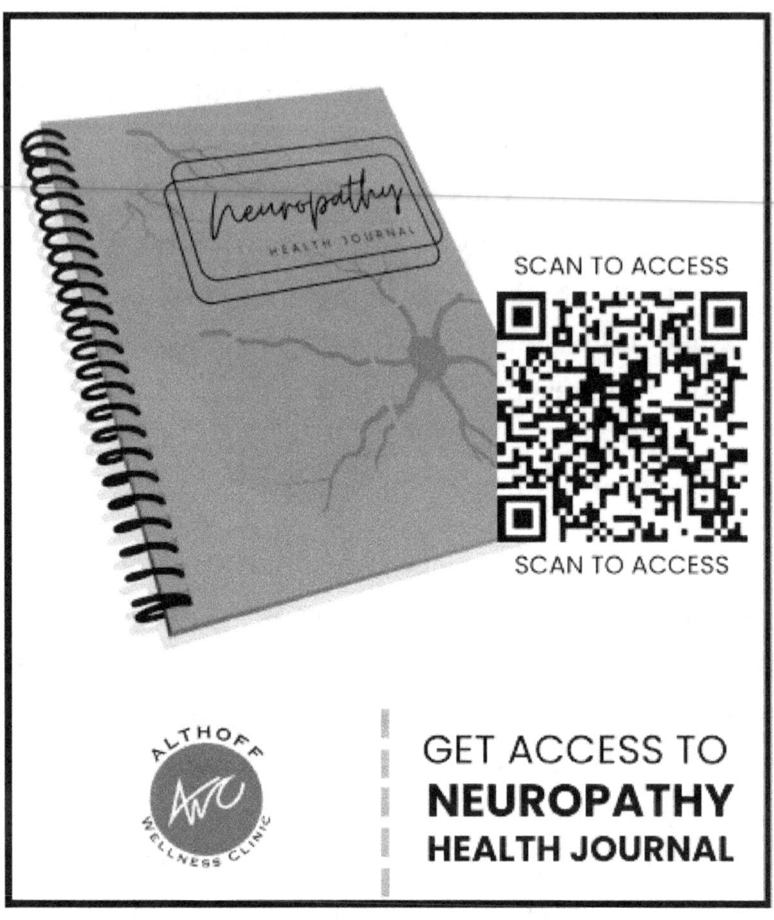

Unlock Your Path to Neuropathy Relief Now: Visit DrJillAlthoff.Com or Call (970) 579-7496 to Speak With Us Today!

Individual results may vary. Please review the disclaimer after the Table of Contents.

2

DO WE HAVE HEALTHCARE OR SICKCARE IN AMERICA?

Modern medicine in America is predominantly crisis-focused, which we like to call "Sickcare." It's a system that allows the average American to burn the candle at both ends for decades, only to rely on quick fixes like open-heart surgery to keep going. This cycle often leads to a retirement marked by exhaustion, disability, and financial strain.

The Dalai Lama once remarked on this paradox: "Man sacrifices his health to make money. Then he sacrifices money to recuperate his health. He is so anxious about the future that he does not enjoy the present; the result being that he does not live in the present or the future; he lives as if he is never going to die, and then dies having never really lived."

Think about it. Are you motivated to be well right now, or will you only be motivated when illness threatens to take away your life? Sadly, many of us only find our motivation when something goes wrong. It's easier to choose cheeseburgers and couch time over healthier choices until a health crisis strikes. These poor lifestyle choices are the root cause of many diseases we face today. We should be motivated every day to live a lifestyle that allows us to thrive, maintain, and enjoy a fantastic quality of life.

Wellness Over Sickcare

Wellness is about seeking health proactively rather than waiting for illness to strike. There's no medication, special lotion, surgery, or injection that can regain your health once it's lost. Modern medicine often operates on the belief that aging is the decline phase of life. We're born, we live, we get sick, and we die. But it doesn't have to be that way.

We need a mindset shift. Instead of viewing our bodies as vessels destined for deterioration, we should see them as capable of continuous progress. Yes, we will all age and eventually die, but imagine how different your life could be if you decided to live up to your physical potential from now on.

Embracing Wellness Care

More people are realizing that focusing on wellness can help them live healthier, longer lives. They are demanding that their healthcare providers work with them on wellness plans that prevent, rather than cure, diseases and pain. Evidence of this shift is all around us: organic and local foods are becoming the preferred produce options in America and around the world. The Veterans Administration is implementing alternative therapies to help veterans deal with pain and avoid opioid addictions. According to Harvard Medical School, Americans make about 425 million visits to holistic health care providers each year.

Part of this Wellness Revolution is a shift in the doctor-patient relationship. People no longer take their doctor's advice as the final word on health concerns. They are more likely to ask questions, seek second opinions, and research alternative treatments. The patient, rather than the doctor, is now the decision-maker in their wellness journey.

The Role of Modern Medicine in Sickcare

Make no mistake, modern medicine plays an important role in our healthcare system. The more open and receptive your primary care physician is to discussing your wellness care, the more of a partner they can become in your ongoing health. Modern healthcare groups all health-related concepts and activities into three categories:

1. **Self-Care:** The daily choices you make about diet, exercise, stress management, and more.
2. **Healthcare:** The proactive steps you take to maintain good health, such as seeking wellness providers, getting educated on fitness and exercise, and participating in wellness programs.
3. **Sickcare (Crisis Care):** The care we seek when disaster strikes. When we get sick or injured, we go to the doctor to fix what we cannot handle on our own. Self-care and healthcare aim to prevent the need for crisis care.

Choosing to stop smoking won't prevent a car accident, but it can significantly reduce your risk of developing cancer, heart attacks, or other conditions. Of course, there will be instances where serious illness or injury necessitates crisis care, but many illnesses are preventable with better lifestyle choices.

America's Sickcare System: A Crash Course in Getting Well

America's current healthcare system promotes drugs and surgery above all else, including prevention. In 2021, American prescription drug spending totaled $378 billion. Despite this spending, America is still getting sicker. The tragedy is that most illnesses requiring crisis care are preventable. There are likely dozens of lifestyle choices you could improve upon.

Here are a few simple suggestions to get you back on track:

- **Get regular moderate exercise:** Physical activity is crucial for heart health, weight management, bone strength, and immune function.
- **Stay well-hydrated:** Water is essential for every bodily function.
- **Eat a plant-based, nutrient-dense diet:** Focus on fruits, vegetables, whole grains, and lean proteins.
- **Get adequate sleep:** Most people need seven to eight hours of sleep each night to function at their best.
- **Avoid harmful habits:** This includes smoking and excessive alcohol consumption.

- **Find healthy ways to manage stress:** Engage in activities and surround yourself with people who boost your mood.
- **Seek support from trusted healthcare practitioners:** Find professionals who can guide you in maintaining your wellness.

The Long-Term Impact of Daily Choices

People often feel conflicted when making lifestyle changes. It's easier to skip the gym, order the cheeseburger, or postpone quitting smoking. These choices may seem insignificant at the moment, but they add up over time. Ten, twenty, thirty years from now, will you regret your lifestyle choices?

The essential question is: How can you improve your current level of functioning? By making small, consistent changes today, you can significantly impact your future health and well-being.

You have a choice?

Which model of health care do you currently embrace? Reflect deeply on your motivations and daily choices. Are you proactive in our wellness journey, or do you wait for a crisis to push you into action? Modern medicine, while indispensable, should ideally complement a robust wellness care regimen. It's crucial to recognize that the choices we make today will shape our health for years to come. Ultimately, the question we must ask ourselves is: how can we improve our current level of functioning? By making small, consistent changes, we can pave the way for a healthier, more vibrant future. Let this chapter be a catalyst for rethinking your approach to health—transforming from a reactive sickcare mindset to a proactive wellness journey. The goal is to thrive, not just survive. Embrace the wellness movement, make proactive choices, and live a life of vibrant health and fulfillment.

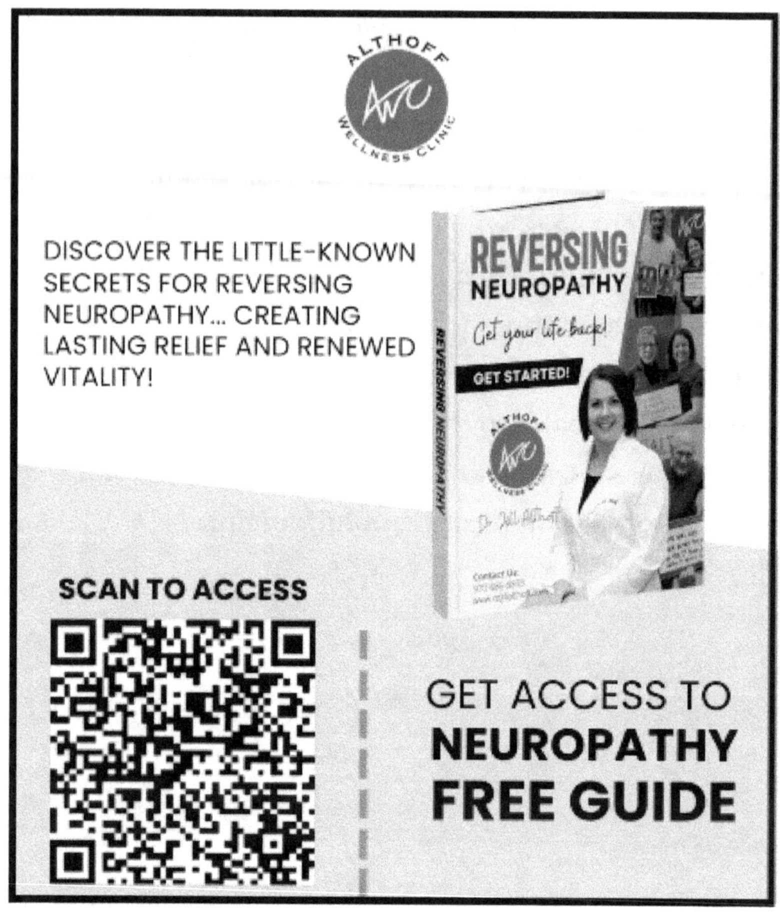

Unlock Your Path to Neuropathy Relief Now: Visit DrJillAlthoff.Com or Call (970) 579-7496 to Speak With Us Today!

Individual results may vary. Please review the disclaimer after the Table of Contents.

3

UNDERSTANDING THE ENEMY: NEUROPATHY

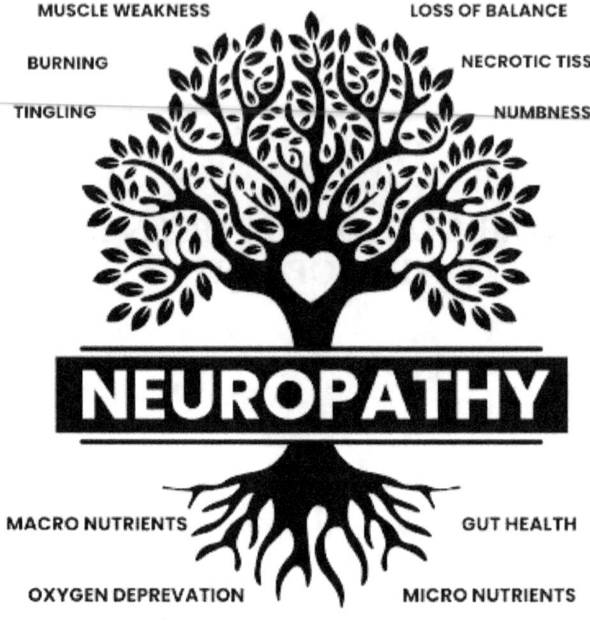

I often see the fear in my patients' eyes when they first tell me about their neuropathy. It's a feeling I understand all too well. The constant pain, the tingling, the numbness—it can feel like a thief, stealing away the simple joys of life. I remember Barbara, a woman who came to me a year ago, her spirit dimmed by the relentless grip of neuropathy. "I could hardly walk, and the pain kept me awake at night," she confessed, her voice heavy with exhaustion. "It made it difficult to do anything."

But Barbara, like many others, found a path to healing with the REPAIR program. She committed to the journey, and slowly but surely, she began to reclaim her life. It was heartwarming to watch her confidence blossom. Just a few months ago, she came in for an appointment with a smile on her face, saying, "I can actually get out and do things now. I can walk without pain, and I'm sleeping through the night! It's like a whole new world."

Of course, every patient's journey is unique, and results can vary. But Barbara's story, like many others, highlights the potential of the REPAIR program to bring meaningful relief and a better quality of life to those struggling with neuropathy.

What is Peripheral Neuropathy?

Peripheral neuropathy affects millions of people worldwide, causing pain, numbness, and tingling in the extremities. This condition can significantly impact one's quality of life, making simple tasks challenging. Understanding what neuropathy is and its underlying causes is the first step toward effective treatment.

Understanding Peripheral Neuropathy

The nervous system is divided into two main parts: the central nervous system and the peripheral nervous system. The central nervous system consists of the brain and spinal cord, acting as the control center for the body. The peripheral nervous system includes all the nerves that branch out from the spinal cord to the rest of the body. These nerves are crucial as they connect the central nervous system to the limbs and organs, affecting every aspect of health. The peripheral nerves extend to the arms, legs, digestive tract, heart, lungs, and more.

Peripheral neuropathy occurs when these peripheral nerves are damaged or disrupted. The most common areas affected are the hands and feet, where patients often experience symptoms first. Imagine your nervous system as a network of highways, with nerves acting as the roads that connect your brain to the rest of your body. Neuropathy disrupts these highways, causing traffic jams and detours. It's like having potholes on your information superhighway, leading to sensations like pins and needles or numbness.

Symptoms and Impact on Daily Life

Peripheral neuropathy can manifest in various ways:

- **Gradual Onset:** It may start with a slight "off" feeling in the fingertips or toes and slowly progress.

- **Sudden Onset:** It can strike suddenly, like a bolt of pain that makes walking feel excruciating.

Peripheral neuropathy can wreak havoc on every aspect of your life. Imagine struggling to button your shirt, type on a keyboard, or even hold a coffee cup without trembling hands. Daily activities like walking the dog, gardening, or cooking dinner can become painful, laborious tasks. Hobbies you once loved, such as playing the piano, painting, or golfing, might feel impossible due to constant numbness, tingling, or burning sensations in your extremities.

The impact extends beyond physical activities. At work, you might find it challenging to focus or complete tasks, leading to decreased productivity and stress. Socially, you might withdraw from friends and family, avoiding gatherings due to discomfort or embarrassment over your condition.

Peripheral neuropathy significantly increases the risk of severe health problems. A minor cut on your foot can escalate into a dangerous ulcer or infection because you can't feel it. The lack of sensation can also lead to frequent falls, causing fractures or other injuries. Moreover, the stress and inactivity resulting from neuropathy can contribute to heart problems, compounding your health issues.

If left untreated, peripheral neuropathy can cause irreversible nerve damage, potentially leading to permanent disability. The thought of losing independence, relying on a walker or wheelchair, or needing constant care can be terrifying. This condition doesn't just take away your ability to function—it steals your quality of life, piece by piece.

Causes of Peripheral Neuropathy

Neuropathy is a complex condition with multiple causes, often interconnected. Here are some of the common contributors:

- **Diabetes:** High blood sugar levels can damage nerves over time, making diabetes one of the leading causes of neuropathy.
- **Blood Sugar Dysregulation:** Even in the absence of diabetes, poor blood sugar control can contribute to nerve damage.
- **Systemic Inflammation:** Chronic inflammation in the body can affect nerve health, leading to neuropathy.
- **Gut Health Issues:** Poor gut health can impact nutrient absorption, which is crucial for nerve function.

- **Nutrient Deficiencies:** Deficiencies in vitamins and minerals, such as B vitamins and magnesium, can impair nerve health.
- **Circulation Issues:** Poor blood flow deprives nerves of essential nutrients and oxygen, leading to damage.
- **Stroke:** A stroke can cause damage to the central nervous system, which may result in peripheral neuropathy.
- **Injury/Trauma:** Physical injuries can damage nerves directly or through the development of scar tissue.
- **Spinal Problems:** Issues with the spine, such as herniated discs or spinal stenosis, can compress nerves and lead to neuropathy.
- **Exposure to Toxins:** Certain toxins, including chemotherapy drugs and heavy metals, can damage nerves. Chemotherapy-induced peripheral neuropathy is a common side effect for many cancer patients. These drugs can be more likely to cause neuropathy when administered frequently or at higher doses.
- **Autoimmune Diseases:** Conditions like lupus, rheumatoid arthritis, and Guillain-Barré syndrome can cause the immune system to attack nerve tissues, leading to neuropathy.

Often, neuropathy is caused by a combination of these factors. Addressing the underlying causes is essential for effective treatment.

The Painful Journey

Stage 1: The Whispers of Discomfort

Neuropathy often starts subtly: a tingling sensation in the toes, clumsiness in the fingers, or fleeting numbness. Patients often describe it as feeling like a sock is bunched up under their foot. Recognizing these early signs is crucial for timely intervention.

Stage 2: Escalating Symptoms

The whispers become shouts. Tingling intensifies into burning pain or a constant ache. Additional symptoms include cramping, poor circulation, cold feet, and physical changes in the feet such as yellowing or fungal nails, color changes, dry skin, and hair loss. Hypersensitivity can also develop, where even a light touch can cause significant pain. Weakness sets in, making it harder to grip objects or walk steadily. Loss of sensation can creep in, leaving you feeling disconnected from your own body.

Stage 3: The Crossroads of Choice

Symptoms become more constant and severe. Wounds and sores are slow to heal, increasing the risk of infections. At this stage, you may need assistance with mobility, such as using a cane or walker, leading to a more sedentary lifestyle. Daily activities become a challenge, and your independence is threatened. Yet, amidst the pain and frustration, a crucial opportunity emerges. Early and appropriate treatment can significantly slow progression and even lead to improvement. This is where our REPAIR neuropathy program steps in, offering a holistic approach to managing and potentially reversing the damage.

Stage 4: Living with Neuropathy

In some cases, neuropathy may reach an advanced stage where symptoms become debilitating. Patients may become dependent on others to complete simple daily activities, such as dressing, bathing, and eating. While it may be possible to reverse some of the neuropathy, it is unlikely that all of it can be reversed. Concerns at this stage also include a higher risk of serious complications such as infections, sepsis, necrosis, gangrene, and amputations. The focus here is on managing symptoms, preventing complications, and maintaining the highest possible quality of life. We'll explore various pain management techniques, assistive devices, and lifestyle modifications to help you navigate this stage with dignity and resilience.

Personal Patient Stories

Hearing personal stories helps us understand the impact of peripheral neuropathy:

Tom's Story: A Loss of Independence

Tom had always been the rock of his family, taking pride in maintaining their yard and home. But neuropathy gradually stole his strength and coordination, leaving him feeling frustrated and useless. "I can't even mow the lawn or help with yard work anymore," Tom shared. "Watching my wife struggle to do everything on her own breaks my heart. It used to be something we enjoyed together, and now I feel like I'm holding her back." The loss of independence and the inability to contribute to his household tasks have taken a significant toll on Tom's sense of pride and self-worth.

Mary's Story: The Emotional Burden

Mary, a dedicated dog lover, cherished her daily walks with her golden retriever, Max. But as neuropathy progressed, the pain and numbness in her feet made walking increasingly difficult. "I can no longer walk Max around the neighborhood," Mary confessed, tears welling up in her eyes. "It's not just about the walk; it's about the connection and joy we both shared. I feel like I'm failing him and myself." The emotional burden of not being able to engage in simple activities with her beloved pet has left Mary feeling isolated and disheartened.

John's Story: A Struggle for Normalcy

John prided himself on being active and involved in his family's life, from playing catch with his grandkids to taking care of household chores. But neuropathy has made even the simplest tasks unbearable. "I used to be the one my family could rely on, but now I feel like a burden," John explained. "I can't help with anything around the house, and watching my loved ones pick up the slack makes me feel so helpless." John's struggle to maintain a sense of normalcy and contribute to his family's daily life has left him feeling disconnected and deeply frustrated.

Neuropathy isn't just about the physical aches and stumbles; it's a thief that can steal away your joy, independence, and peace of mind. Let's talk about the emotional and physical costs this condition can create.

Emotional and Psychological Impact:

- Loss of Independence. Patients may feel a sense of helplessness and dependence on others, leading to decreased self-esteem and self-worth.
- Social Isolation. Reduced ability to engage in social activities can lead to loneliness and social withdrawal.
- Depression and Anxiety. Chronic pain and the inability to perform daily activities can contribute to mental health issues, including depression and anxiety.
- Frustration and Anger. Struggling with simple tasks can cause frustration and anger, impacting relationships with family and friends.

Financial Impact:

- Medical Costs. Continuous treatment and medications for neuropathy can be financially draining.
- Home Modifications. Modifying the home to accommodate mobility issues can be costly.
- Loss of Income. Inability to work or reduced

working hours can lead to a significant loss of income.

Quality of Life:

- Reduced Physical Activity. Inability to stay active can lead to further health complications, such as obesity and heart disease.
- Limitations on Hobbies and Interests. Inability to engage in hobbies and activities that once brought joy can diminish overall life satisfaction.

Navigating with Coping Strategies

Neuropathy can be challenging, but effective coping strategies can help you manage the condition and improve your quality of life:

- **The Power of Perspective:** Shift your mindset from "I am a victim" to "I am a warrior." This empowers you to take control and become an active participant in your own healing journey.
- **Finding Your Support System:** Lean on loved ones, join support groups, or seek professional therapy. Sharing experiences and learning from others can be a powerful source of strength and inspiration.

- **Nourishing Your Body and Mind:** Embrace a nutrient-rich diet and engage in gentle exercises. Prioritize rest and incorporate stress-management techniques like yoga or meditation. Self-care is a necessity in this battle.
- **Celebrating Small Victories:** Acknowledge even the smallest achievements. Celebrating progress, no matter how small, fuels your motivation and keeps you moving forward.

The Red Flags of Neuropathy Emergencies

Understanding the signs that indicate a neuropathy emergency is crucial for timely intervention:

- **Rapidly Worsening Pain:** Imagine the familiar discomfort suddenly amplifying to a level that steals your breath and renders daily activities impossible. This drastic escalation in pain can be a sign of nerve damage reaching a critical point, requiring immediate medical attention.
- **Loss of Sensory Perception:** When numbness takes over, not just tingling, but a complete absence of feeling in your legs or feet, it's a serious red flag. This can make you unaware of

injuries, increasing the risk of burns, cuts, and infections.

- **Motor Function Decline:** Stumbling becomes frequent falls, gripping objects feels impossible, and simple movements demand immense effort. This rapid decline in motor skills indicates potential nerve damage in crucial areas, necessitating urgent intervention.
- **Bladder and Bowel Dysfunction:** When neuropathy disrupts the delicate messages between your nerves and your bladder or bowel, it can lead to sudden loss of control or difficulty with urination or bowel movements. These changes require immediate medical evaluation to prevent complications.
- **Autonomic System Disruption:** In rare cases, neuropathy can affect the autonomic nervous system, which controls involuntary functions like heart rate, blood pressure, and sweating. This can lead to life-threatening situations like rapid heart rate changes or difficulty breathing, requiring immediate emergency care.

By understanding the nature of neuropathy, recognizing the symptoms, and identifying the causes, you are taking the first step towards managing this condition. In the following chapters, we will dive deeper into the holistic and integrative approaches that can help you reclaim your quality of life and manage neuropathy effectively.

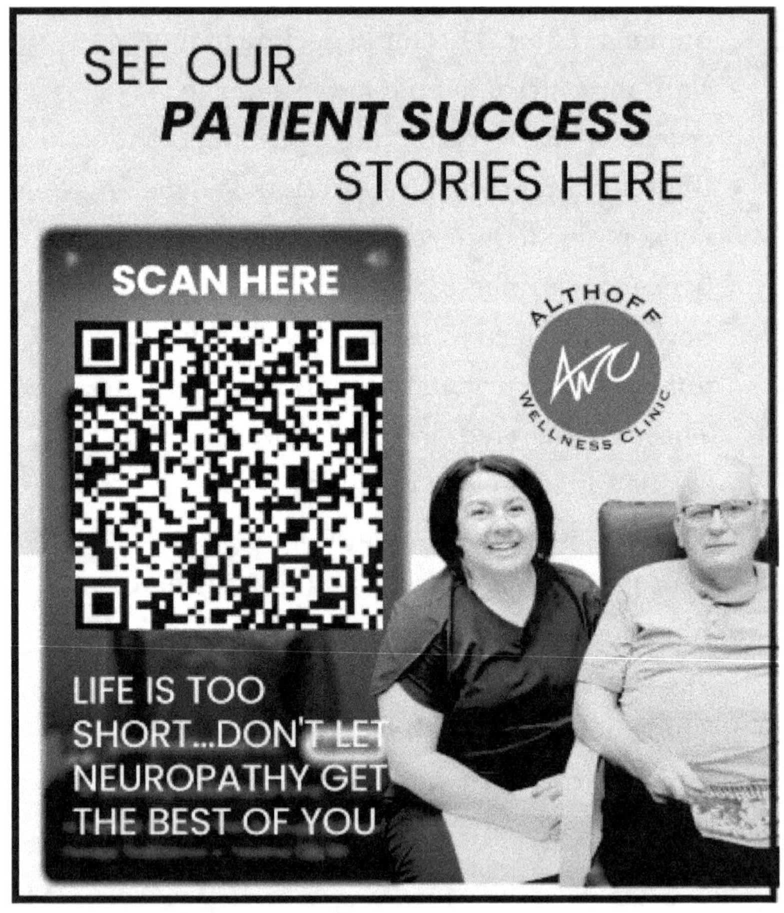

Unlock Your Path to Neuropathy Relief Now: Visit DrJillAlthoff.Com or Call (970) 579-7496 to Speak With Us Today!

Individual results may vary. Please review the disclaimer after the Table of Contents.

4

———

NEUROPATHY MYTHS: SEPARATING FACT FROM FICTION

Fear and uncertainty often accompany neuropathy. Amidst the fog of information, myths and misconceptions can make the path to healing even more confusing. Let's shed light on some common myths, turning them into stepping stones on your journey to well-being.

Myth 1: Nerve damage is irreversible.

Reality: Nerve damage can often be reversed or slowed down, depending on the cause, duration, and severity. Think about when you've had surgery with an incision. Oftentimes, the area around the incision is numb right after the surgery. But over time, you regain some of that feeling. Why? Because the sensory nerves repair themselves. Given the right conditions, such as proper nutrients and care, nerves can regenerate. Treatments like regenerative medicine, vitamin therapy, nerve stimulation, and alternative therapies such as acupuncture and massage can stimulate nerve growth and repair. However, effectiveness varies, and it's important to consult a neuropathy specialist before trying any treatment.

Many patients spend hundreds of dollars on devices off the internet that claim to heal nerve damage, but most of these devices are gimmicks. Additionally, some patients take supplements from unreliable sources that claim to help neuropathy but end up creating more toxins in the body, delaying healing or even worsening the condition. Always seek professional advice before trying new treatments to ensure safety and efficacy.

Myth 2: Only people with diabetes develop neuropathy.

Reality: While diabetes is a common cause (approximately 40% of our patients suffer from diabetes), neuropathy can stem from various sources, including infections, injuries, toxins, inherited disorders, and idiopathic causes (unknown origins). 60-70% of diabetics suffer from peripheral neuropathy. However, anyone can develop neuropathy, regardless of whether they have diabetes. Recognizing the signs and seeking medical help is crucial for early intervention.

Myth 3: Prescription medications cure neuropathy.

Reality: Prescription medications treat the symptoms but do not address the root cause of neuropathy. Unfortunately, they often do not manage the symptoms all that well either. These medications may provide temporary relief but fail to tackle the underlying nerve damage. Additionally, they can have side effects like drowsiness, dementia, nausea, weight gain, and addiction. Exploring other treatment options that address the root cause of neuropathy is essential for long-term relief.

Myth 4: Tingling, numbness, and shooting pains are the only symptoms of neuropathy.

Reality: Tingling, numbness, and shooting pains are the only symptoms of neuropathy. Reality: Neuropathy symptoms can vary widely, including burning pain, cold hands and feet, restless leg syndrome, and cramping. Additionally, symptoms can encompass weakness, balance and coordination problems, organ issues, and changes in sensitivity. These symptoms can be mild or severe and can affect one or multiple parts of the body. Being aware of the diverse symptoms and reporting any changes to your doctor is crucial for proper diagnosis and treatment.

Myth 5: Neuropathy has no cure.

Reality: While challenging, neuropathy is not hopeless. Treatment depends on the cause, type, and severity of nerve damage and aims to prevent further damage, relieve symptoms, and stimulate nerve growth or repair. Success requires realistic expectations, time, and patient dedication and commitment. Significant improvements are possible with the right approach.

Unveiling the Truth: Overcoming Neuropathy Treatment Myths

"Knowledge is power," especially true when navigating the often-murky waters of neuropathy treatment. Misinformation can delay effective treatment, create unrealistic expectations, breed fear and anxiety, and promote harmful practices. Let's explore how to navigate this maze with critical thinking and credible information.

The Dangers of Misinformation:

- **Delays Effective Treatment:** Clinging to myths can prevent proper diagnosis and evidence-based treatment, allowing neuropathy to progress.

- **Fuels Unrealistic Expectations:** False promises of miracle cures can lead to disappointment and hinder progress.
- **Breeds Fear and Anxiety:** Misinformation can make you feel powerless and trapped, exacerbating pain and affecting mental well-being.
- **Promotes Harmful Practices:** Desperation can lead to unproven, potentially dangerous treatments.

How to Navigate and Master the Maze:

- **Be a Skeptical Sherlock:** Question sources, research claims, and consult qualified healthcare professionals.
- **Embrace Evidence-Based Sources:** Stick to reputable medical websites, research papers, and established institutions like Mayo Clinic, MedlinePlus, and the National Institute of Health. Seek guidance from certified specialists.
- **Listen to Your Body:** Pay attention to its signals, track progress, and be honest with your healthcare team about what works and what hasn't.

- **Join the Support Tribe:** Connect with others living with neuropathy to share experiences, resources, and learn from each other's journeys.

The Path to Clarity: Discerning Facts in Neuropathy Treatment

Developing critical thinking and evaluating information is crucial in discerning fact from fiction. Here are essential tools to help you identify truths in neuropathy treatment:

1. Source Validation:

- **Credibility Check:** Ensure information comes from qualified professionals or reputable institutions.
- **Bias Assessment:** Be wary of sources pushing specific agendas or products.

2. Evidence-Based Evaluation:

- **Scientific Backing:** Look for claims supported by reputable research and published in peer-reviewed journals.
- **Logical Consistency:** Ensure information

aligns with established medical knowledge and principles.

3. Contextualization:

- **Individualization:** Recognize that everyone's experience with neuropathy is unique. Individual factors must be considered.
- **Long-Term Perspective:** Be skeptical of quick fixes and focus on comprehensive, long-term approaches.

4. Professional Consultation:

- **Seek Expert Guidance:** Consult with qualified healthcare professionals for personalized advice.
- **Second Opinions:** Don't hesitate to seek second opinions for a broader perspective on your treatment plan.

Identifying truths in neuropathy treatment requires skepticism and a commitment to critical thinking. By following these guidelines and seeking professional advice, you can confidently navigate the labyrinth of information and find the most effective treatment options for your needs.

Robin's Journey: From Fear to Freedom

Robin came to Althoff Wellness Clinic PC with a heart heavy with worry. Neuropathy had invaded her body, bringing with it a relentless wave of numbness in her hands and feet. "It was so bad," Robin recalls, her voice tinged with the memory of those difficult days. "Walking was incredibly painful, things would constantly fall out of my hands, and I felt utterly exhausted all the time."

The numbness extended beyond her physical sensations; it had begun to numb her spirit. "I was terrified," Robin confesses, "I truly believed I might lose my right foot. Every doctor I saw reinforced that fear, telling me there was nothing I could do except try to manage the pain and accept my fate."

Robin's neuropathy was affecting every aspect of her life. Her days were clouded by fatigue, and her once-vibrant spirit felt dimmed. "I couldn't keep up with my husband," she shares, "He's incredibly active, and it was heartbreaking to feel like I was holding him back." The thought of a future where she couldn't participate in life to the fullest filled her with despair.

Then Robin discovered Althoff Wellness Clinic PC and the REPAIR program. It was a leap of faith, a decision born out of a desperate longing for a different path. "I knew it was going to be a lot of work," Robin says, "but after hearing Dr. Althoff's explanation of the program and feeling the genuine care from the entire staff, I decided to embrace the opportunity."

A year later, Robin's life is a testament to the power of hope and a personalized approach. "The changes have been incredible," she shares, her eyes shining. "I'm sleeping better, my energy has returned, and I can keep up with my husband again!" But the most profound victory for Robin is the return of feeling to her feet. "My recent nerve conduction test showed that the neuropathy in my feet has reduced to under 15%!" she exclaims, a triumphant smile lighting up her face. "I can walk without pain, and the fear of losing my foot is finally gone."

Success with this program is not guaranteed for everyone, but Robin's journey reminds us that healing is possible, even when faced with seemingly insurmountable obstacles. Her story reinforces the core message of this chapter: don't let the fog of misinformation steal your hope. By embracing knowledge, seeking evidence-based solutions, and trusting in your body's innate capacity to heal, you can navigate the complexities of neuropathy and reclaim a life filled with possibility.

ACTION STEP: Take our free Nerve Damage Evaluation by scanning this code:

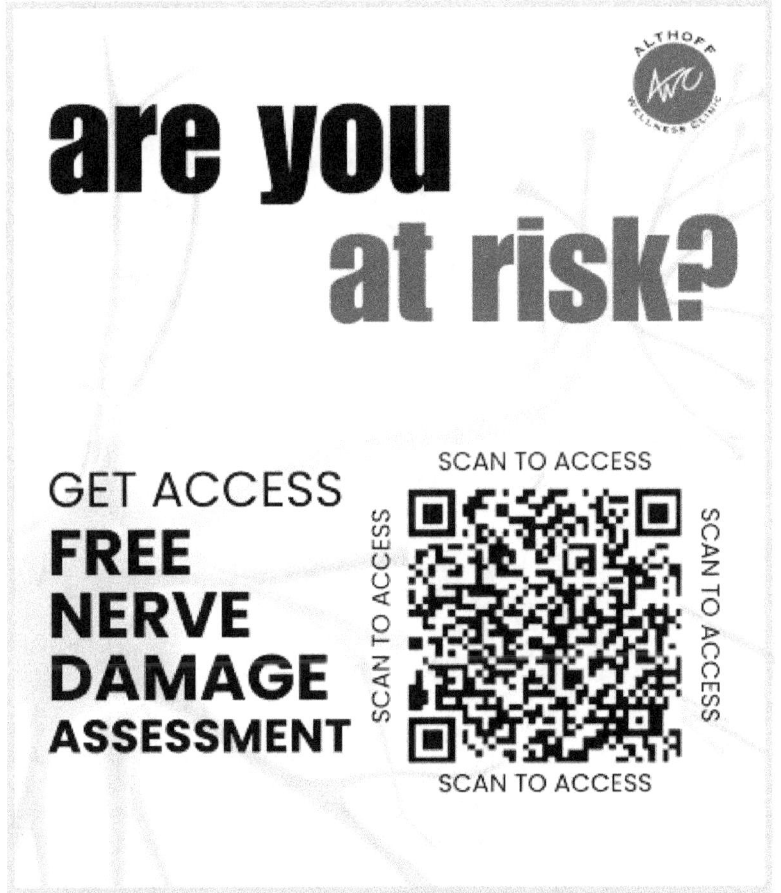

Unlock Your Path to Neuropathy Relief Now: Visit DrJillAlthoff.Com or Call (970) 579-7496 to Speak With Us Today!

Individual results may vary. Please review the disclaimer after the Table of Contents.

REPAIR: YOUR ROADMAP TO NERVE HEALING

Living with neuropathy can feel like a constant struggle, where even the simplest tasks become burdensome. The REPAIR Neuropathy Program is here to guide you through this journey, offering a structured and effective path to regain your health and well-being. Each step of the REPAIR program is designed to address different aspects of neuropathy and provide you with the tools and support needed for lasting recovery.

In this chapter, we embark on a critical exploration: understanding the powerful connection between lifestyle choices and the development and management of peripheral neuropathy. The REPAIR program rests on this very foundation, recognizing that diet, exercise, and stress management each play a crucial role in your nerve health journey.

Think of your body as a complex ecosystem and your nerves as vital pathways coursing through it. Lifestyle factors are the environmental elements – the sun, rain, and soil – that nourish or neglect these pathways. An imbalance in this ecosystem, such as excessive sugar intake, sedentary habits, or chronic stress, can weaken your nerves, creating fertile ground for neuropathy to develop.

But here's the empowering truth: the REPAIR neuropathy program empowers you to become the architect of your own nerve health. Let's dissect the acronym, each letter representing a fundamental principle in your journey:

R – Root Cause Discovery

The R in REPAIR marks a crucial starting point in our journey: uncovering the precise cause of your neuropathy. Often this involves identifying underlying factors that can be easily overlooked; vitamin deficiencies, hidden toxins, chronic stress, poor circulation and oxygenation just to name a few. This is not about pointing fingers or assigning blame; it's about gaining critical insight to unlock targeted interventions and optimize your path to nerve health. This allows for development of a personalized treatment plan that targets the source of your symptoms rather than just addressing the symptoms themselves.

At Althoff Wellness Clinic PC, a leading chiropractic clinic in Windsor, Colorado and Cheyenne, Wyoming, we go above and beyond with our comprehensive testing approach. Alongside the detailed medical history, complete physical exam, and specific diagnostic tests, we perform a meticulous 16-point nerve examination. Our thorough evaluation includes an in-depth analysis of your blood flow and oxygen levels. Our team also assesses your motor nervous system to determine any impacts. Additionally, we delve into your diet and inflammatory response, conducting a very thorough consultation to uncover any pertinent history contributing to your neuropathy.

Common root causes include diabetes, toxins, autoimmune conditions, stroke, trauma, chemotherapy, and spinal-related issues. Often, it is a combination of these factors. Each piece of evidence gathered adds another brushstroke to the picture. Perhaps your neuropathy stems from the metabolic imbalances associated with diabetes, requiring focused interventions on blood sugar management. Or maybe a silent vitamin B12 deficiency is depriving your nerves of essential nutrients, necessitating targeted supplementation. In some cases, an underlying autoimmune condition might be playing a role, demanding tailored therapies and lifestyle modifications to address the root cause.

Once the root cause is uncovered personalization of your REPAIR program begins. For diabetes, a plan is crafted rich in dietary adjustments, exercise strategies, and blood sugar management tools. For a B12 deficiency, specific supplementation is prescribed to nourish the nerves. In the face of an autoimmune battleground, individualized interventions are developed to restore, balance, and protect nerve pathways.

Every case is unique, and Althoff Wellness Clinic takes pride in treating each patient individually with programs tailored to their specific needs. This is a crucial step that other clinics overlook or miss, leading to lack of outcomes and patient success.

E – Eliminate Contributing Factors

The E in REPAIR signifies a crucial transition from merely identifying the root cause of your neuropathy to actively reducing its impact. Our goal is to pinpoint and eliminate the modifiable risk factors that contribute to neuropathy, creating a strong foundation for nerve healing and overall health. This may involve dietary changes, stress management techniques, or gentle electrohydraulic technology. Here is where we shed the gardener's analytical cap and don the proactive gloves of elimination.

E focuses on removing the weeds – dietary imbalances, sedentary habits, chronic stress, and harmful toxins – that further impede optimal functioning. Each harmful element removed strengthens your body's innate defense mechanisms against neuropathy.

This is where collaboration takes center stage. We'll work together to develop personalized strategies for:

- Optimizing Dietary Intake: We'll delve into the world of nerve-supportive nutrition, swapping sugary weeds for vibrant blooms of colorful vegetables, juicy fruits, and whole grains. We'll prioritize low-glycemic delights that stabilize blood sugar levels, preventing damaging spikes that weaken your nerves. Think leafy greens, berries, melons, nuts, and whole grains – a symphony of deliciousness that nourishes your nerves and strengthens your defenses. Additionally, we may eliminate foods that cause high inflammation, such as sugar, simple carbs, dairy, and sometimes even nightshades and oxidative foods.

- **Deliciously Nutritious Food:** We ditch the concept of restrictive diets and embrace the joy of vibrant, nerve-nourishing meals. Think colorful salads, juicy berries, whole grains, and lean protein – a variety of flavors that fuels your body and delights your taste buds. We'll create personalized strategies to overcome cravings and make healthy choices the easy, delicious, and sustainable option.
- Eliminating Toxins: We'll also focus on reducing or eliminating toxins like alcohol and smoking, which can exacerbate nerve damage and inflammation. Furthermore, we may eliminate potential parasites and heavy metals from the system using gentle detox methods.
- Embracing Regular Physical Activity: Physical activity isn't just about sculpted physiques; it's a potent tonic for nerve health. We'll uncover an enjoyable activity that resonates with you, whether gentle yoga, brisk walks in nature, or even dancing in your living room. Each movement becomes a vital raindrop watering your nerve garden, flushing out toxins, and boosting overall well-being.
- **Movement that Makes You Move:** Physical activity isn't about grueling workouts; it's about finding joy in movement. We'll explore

activities you genuinely enjoy, be it brisk walks in nature, dancing in your living room, or joining a gentle yoga class. Remember, consistency is key; small, regular movements become the bricks on which your castle of well-being is built.

- Managing Stress Effectively: Chronic stress can wreak havoc on your nerves. We have potent antidotes! We'll explore evidence-based stress management techniques like meditation and deep breathing, helping you cultivate inner peace and silence the stressful chorus.

- **Calming the Stressful Tides:** Chronic stress is the enemy within, but 'I' equips you with the tools to combat it. We'll explore mindfulness techniques like meditation and deep breathing and practical strategies for managing daily stressors. Imagine these techniques as soothing waves washing over your mind, calming the tempest, and creating a haven for your nervous system to thrive.

Imagine soothing music washing over your garden, calming the frenzy, and creating a haven for your nerves to thrive. With every healthy bite, every mindful movement, and every controlled breath, you strengthen your body's natural defenses against neuropathy and pave the way for a future where your nerves sing in harmonious well-being.

P – Pain Relief

Pain relief is a critical component of the REPAIR program. P marks a shift from identifying the enemy to alleviating its immediate influence through pain relief. While we diligently work towards long-term healing by addressing the root cause of your neuropathy, your present comfort remains our paramount concern. We offer a variety of natural pain management strategies to help with the discomfort of neuropathy. This includes soothing herbs, targeted stretches, mindfulness techniques, and gentle movement practices. Our goal is to equip you with effective methods to manage pain and improve your quality of life. Experiencing unnecessary pain shouldn't be a part of your journey to reclaim your life.

Our pain management arsenal is vast and evidence-based, offering a powerful array of options to suit your unique needs:

- **Nerve Stimulation & Rebuilding:** Utilizing a state-of-the-art electrical stimulation device, this at-home therapy revitalizes nerve function by opening nerve pathways, re-educating nerves, and re-mineralizing synaptic junctions. It offers comprehensive care for the entire nervous system, significantly reducing symptoms like pain and numbness.

- **Light Therapy (LLLT):** Harnesses the power of both infrared and red light, delivering 10,000 mW or 60 Joules per minute. It stimulates the release of nitric oxide, crucial for increasing local blood flow and stimulating new blood vessels. Focused light effectively reduces swelling, alleviates pain, and stimulates healing.

- **SoftWave Tissue Regenerative Technology (TRT):** Known as the 'Stem Cell Machine,' this technology uses acoustic waves to penetrate and rejuvenate injured tissues at a cellular level. It enhances blood circulation, provides vital nutrients and oxygen, and significantly reduces acute and chronic pain. With the ability to stimulate stem cell production this machine introduces a new era in natural regeneration and repair.

- **Class IV Laser Therapy:** Non-invasive, drug-free treatment for neuropathy that uses low-level light energy to stimulate nerve function and promote healing. It penetrates deep into tissues to increase cellular energy, improve circulation, and regenerate tissue. This therapy enhances blood flow, oxygen delivery, and ATP production, which aids in repairing damaged nerve cells. It also helps reduce inflammation, swelling, and pain. Sessions are painless and typically last less than 7 minutes.

- **pEMF (Pulsed Electromagnetic Field):** pEMF therapy stimulates cellular repair and regeneration, effectively reducing neuropathic pain and inflammation and promoting nerve repair. This therapy involves comfortably sitting in a chair while the treatment is administered, making it a non-invasive and relaxing option. Pulsed PEMF therapy treats your cells like batteries, recharging them and amplifying your natural energy to encourage your body to function more effectively. This therapy sends magnetic energy into the body, working with your natural magnetic field to improve healing by increasing electrolytes and ions. It influences electrical changes on a cellular level and helps realign the electricity in your cells, promoting overall wellness and alleviating pain.

- **Neuromed:** NeuroMed's Electroanalgesia (EA) therapy is a non-surgical, drug-free treatment that uses electrical stimulation to alleviate neuropathy pain. It works by stimulating peripheral nerves to block pain messages sent to the brain, providing significant pain relief. Additionally, electrical pulses improve blood circulation, which aids in healing and maintaining nerve tissue. This therapy is effective for managing chronic pain and treating various neuropathy symptoms, such as numbness, tingling, sensitivity to touch, lack of coordination, sharp or burning pain, and muscle weakness. The FDA-cleared NeuroMed system utilizes advanced software and high-frequency signals to deliver precise and effective treatment.

Althoff Wellness Clinic stands out from other surrounding clinics with its arsenal of advanced medical equipment and comprehensive approach to patient care. Our cutting-edge technologies work together to create a comprehensive approach that improves patient outcomes, promoting natural healing and well-being for those experiencing neuropathy. This integrative approach, combined with personalized at-home care and nutritional guidance, ensures our patients receive the most effective, non-invasive, and holistic treatment available.

A – Activate Healing

Your body has an incredible capacity for self-repair, and our program aims to activate this potential. We've cleared the weeds, nurtured the soil, and built bridges, but now, it's time to activate the sunshine, the lifeblood that will spark vibrant growth. Through targeted exercises, nerve-nourishing foods, and mind-body practices such as yoga and meditation, we work to stimulate your body's natural healing processes. A deploys a potent arsenal of tools to nourish and awaken your nerves' inherent healing mechanisms. This holistic approach ensures that your nerves have the support they need to recover and thrive. While targeted nutrients and supplements are important, some of the equipment mentioned above also play a crucial role in activating healing:

- **Targeted Nutrients:** We delve into the world of micronutrient magic, identifying specific vitamins, minerals, and antioxidants that your nerves crave. Imagine Vitamin B12 as a potent fertilizer, revitalizing nerve pathways. Think of Alpha-Lipoic Acid as a gentle rain shower, flushing away toxins and nourishing growth. We'll personalize your nutritional plan, ensuring your nerves receive the precise cocktail of nutrients they need to thrive.

- **Specific Supplements:** Sometimes, your garden needs a little extra boost. We'll explore evidence-based supplements like Omega-3 fatty acids, curcumin, and N-acetylcysteine, each offering unique properties to support nerve repair and regeneration. Think of these supplements as targeted boosters, amplifying your body's innate healing potential.

- **Nerve-Nourishing Practices:** Your body is not just a physical landscape; it's a symphony of mind and movement. We'll introduce gentle yoga postures, mindful meditation practices, and even specific breathing exercises that stimulate nerve function and promote healing. Imagine deep, rhythmic breaths like waves gently rocking your nerve pathways, carrying nutrients and soothing inflammation.

- **Light Therapy (LLLT):** Beyond pain relief, LLLT increases angiogenesis (the formation of new blood capillaries), enhancing blood flow and supporting the healing process.

- **SoftWave Tissue Regenerative Technology (TRT):** This technology not only alleviates pain but also activates stem cells, which significantly boost the body's natural healing capabilities.

- **Class IV Laser Therapy:** The laser improves circulation and activates the healing cycle, ensuring that affected tissues receive the necessary nutrients and oxygen for repair.
- **pEMF (Pulsed Electromagnetic Field):** pEMF therapy increases healing capabilities by stimulating cellular repair and regeneration.

I – Improve Lifestyle

We've alleviated suffering, awakened healing, and now it's time to craft sustainable habits. Because healing extends beyond the treatment room and into your everyday life, making lifestyle improvements that support your overall health and well-being are crucial. As previously mentioned, healthy eating, regular exercise, and effective stress management are the cornerstones of long-term nerve health, however, additional examples include creating a sleep-friendly environment, building supportive relationships, and finding joy and purpose beyond the limitations of neuropathy. These changes are essential for maintaining long-term health and preventing future setbacks. This is where collaboration truly shines. We'll work together to design sustainable, enjoyable habits that fit seamlessly into your life, replacing short-term fixes with permanent transformations:

· Creating a Sleep-Friendly Environment:

Optimize Your Sleep Space: Ensure your bedroom is cool, dark, and quiet. Invest in a comfortable mattress and pillows that support your spine and joints and consider blackout curtains to block out light. Use a white noise machine or earplugs if noise is an issue.

Establish a Pre-Sleep Routine: Develop a calming bedtime routine to signal your body that it's time to wind down. This can include activities like reading a book, taking a warm bath, or practicing gentle stretching or meditation to relax your muscles and mind.

Limit Screen Time: Reduce exposure to screens at least an hour before bedtime, as the blue light emitted can interfere with your body's natural sleep-wake cycle. Instead, engage in relaxing activities that prepare your mind for rest.

· Building Supportive Relationships

Communicate Openly: Share your experiences and feelings about living with neuropathy with friends and family. Open communication fosters understanding and support, allowing your loved ones to offer the help you need.

Join Support Groups: Connect with others who are facing similar challenges by joining neuropathy support groups, either in-person or online. These communities provide a platform to share advice, find encouragement, and build meaningful connections.

Cultivate Positive Relationships: Surround yourself with positive, empathetic individuals who encourage and uplift you. Prioritize relationships that bring joy and understanding, and don't hesitate to seek professional guidance if needed to navigate complex dynamics.

· **Finding Joy and Purpose Beyond the Limitations of Neuropathy**

Pursue Passion Projects: Engage in activities that bring you joy and fulfillment, whether it's a hobby, volunteer work, or learning a new skill. Focusing on what you love can provide a sense of purpose and satisfaction.

Set Achievable Goals: Break down larger aspirations into smaller, manageable steps. Celebrate your progress and accomplishments, no matter how small, to maintain motivation and a positive outlook.

Practice Mindfulness and Gratitude: Incorporate mindfulness practices such as meditation or yoga into your daily routine to stay present and reduce stress. Keeping a gratitude journal can help you focus on the positive aspects of your life and foster a sense of contentment.

R – Retain Results

Our focus is to provide you with tools and strategies to sustain your improvements, prevent relapses, and celebrate each victory along the way. Healing is a continuous process, and it's important to retain the progress you've made, and continue to achieve lasting well-being and a higher quality of life. The final R in REPAIR marks not an ending but a beautiful beginning – embracing lasting resilience and securing your flourishing nerve oasis. By now, you've built a formidable castle of well-being, nurtured from the seeds of healthy habits, and weathered the storms of setbacks. But true mastery lies in safeguarding your progress and thriving not just today, but in the future that awaits.

Here's how we'll ensure your continued success:

- **Knowledge is Power:** We'll delve deeper into the science of neuropathy, empowering you to understand the "whys" and "hows" of your journey. This knowledge becomes your shield, allowing you to navigate challenges with informed choices and proactive measures.

- **Your Support Network:** You're not alone in this endeavor. We'll connect you with a dedicated support network – from healthcare professionals to fellow neuropathy warriors – creating a community of encouragement and shared wisdom. Imagine this network as a vigilant watchtower, always ready to offer guidance and celebrate your victories along the way.

- **Tools for Every Season:** Life is dynamic, and so are your needs. We'll equip you with a flexible toolbox of resources and strategies to adapt to changing circumstances. Think of these tools as weatherproof instruments, allowing you to adjust your sails and navigate unforeseen storms with confidence.

· 1. **Continued Use of Home Care Devices:** You've worked extremely hard to get to where you are, and though the heavy lifting is done, occasional homework is still involved. Our team will ensure recommendations are made regarding utilization of the provided home care devices for continued success and maintaining progress. Frequency of use may vary as every case is unique, however guidance will be provided.

· 2. **Nutritional Guidance and Supplementation:** Upon completion of the program, we offer comprehensive supplement review and consultation. Our AWC Essential Supplements are a great option. Supplements and nutritional products are available to you for purchase upon completion of the program and are very beneficial, such as those aimed at reducing systemic inflammation. Educating patients on the importance of an anti-inflammatory diet and ensuring they understand how specific supplements can support their neuropathy treatment can lead to better long-term outcomes.

· **3. Regular Follow-Up and Progress Monitoring Available:** Even if you've graduated from the program, appointments can be made to re-examine and monitor progress. Ask about a structured follow-up schedule to monitor your progress and make any necessary adjustments to your treatment plan. Regular check-ins, allow for timely modifications and provide patients with ongoing support and encouragement, enhancing their commitment to the program.

· **4. Maintenance Care:** Achieving optimal lasting results with our neuropathy program requires a commitment to ongoing maintenance care. This involves scheduling regular visits to our clinic for periodic assessments and treatments, ensuring any emerging issues are promptly addressed. By staying proactive and vigilant in your health regimen, you can sustain the progress made during the initial phases of the program, prevent relapses, and continue to improve their overall quality of life. Our dedicated team is here to support and guide patients every step of the way, ensuring you remain on the path to optimal health.

Retaining results is not a passive endeavor; it's an ongoing dance of self-awareness, proactive choices, and embracing resilience. We'll be your trusted partners in this dance, celebrating your triumphs, providing unwavering support, and equipping you with the knowledge and tools to navigate any challenge that arises.

The REPAIR program is a personalized journey tailored to your specific needs. We are committed to walking this path with you, providing support and celebrating your successes. With the REPAIR program as your guide, you can navigate the challenges of neuropathy, reclaim your health, and enjoy a fulfilling life.

Rayna's Story: How She Regained Her Balance and Confidence with the REPAIR Neuropathy Program

At Althoff Wellness Clinic PC, we are committed to helping our patients regain control of their lives. One such patient is Rayna, who came to us six months ago with peripheral neuropathy. She struggled with balance, aches, pains, and a lack of awareness in her feet. It was as if she was walking on posts, compensating for the loss of feeling that had gradually crept up on her over time.

After six months of dedicated care under REPAIR, Rayna's transformation has been remarkable. She now feels a renewed connection between her feet, her core, and the ground beneath her. Her balance has improved significantly, enabling her to easily perform daily tasks, like getting dressed without support. Even the small things many of us take for granted have become a testament to her regained power and control.

Rayna's love for underwater exercise has been rekindled, as she can now balance through an entire class, a feat that was previously challenging due to her condition. She no longer has to be cautious about the weights she uses for fear of losing her balance. Instead, she powers through each session with newfound strength and confidence.

Craig's Story: How He Got Back to Golfing with the REPAIR Neuropathy Program

Craig is one of our inspiring patients living with neuropathy since 2002. His neuropathy was getting worse over time, and it was affecting his daily activities and quality of life.

He couldn't walk without pain, he couldn't sleep well, and he couldn't enjoy his favorite hobby, golf. He tried different tests and treatments for his neuropathy, but nothing worked. He was even told by another doctor that he needed surgery, but he didn't want to go that route.

Craig came to our clinic a year ago, looking for a natural and effective solution for his neuropathy. He enrolled in the REPAIR Neuropathy Program, a proven system that combines advanced technology, natural therapies, and lifestyle changes to heal the nerves and improve quality of life. Craig followed the program faithfully for a year, and the results were incredible.

Craig says he feels 80% better than where he started and can walk and balance better. He says his pain is gone, his sleep is better, and his golf game is better. He also says he is optimistic about his future and will continue doing what he's been doing because it's working.

Reclaiming Life: Candy's Journey to Wellness with Althoff Wellness Clinic PC

We believe in the power of alternative care and its potential to transform lives, and our patient, Candy, is a testament to this belief.

When Candy first came to us, she was skeptical. She was suffering from neuropathy, experiencing sleepless nights, constant pain, and a burning sensation that hindered her from enjoying life's simple pleasures. Walking for extended periods was a challenge, and she felt she had lost many of her daily life functions.

However, Candy was determined. She didn't want to rely on medications and sought an alternative care route. That's when she began the REPAIR Neuropathy Program at our clinic.

In just 90 days, Candy's life changed dramatically. The program didn't just alleviate her symptoms; it woke up the nerves in her leg. She now sleeps peacefully at night, no longer needing creams or CBD oil.

Candy takes no medications and can walk for long periods, enjoying precious moments with her grandchildren. She can stand in the kitchen for more than just 10 minutes without any pain, a significant improvement from her initial condition.

These stories are powerful reminders of why we do what we do at Althoff Wellness. If you're struggling with similar issues, we encourage you to reach out. Like our patients, your case could be one we can help transform. Together, we can work towards getting your life back.

** The results described in these testimonials are not typical. Individual results may vary.*

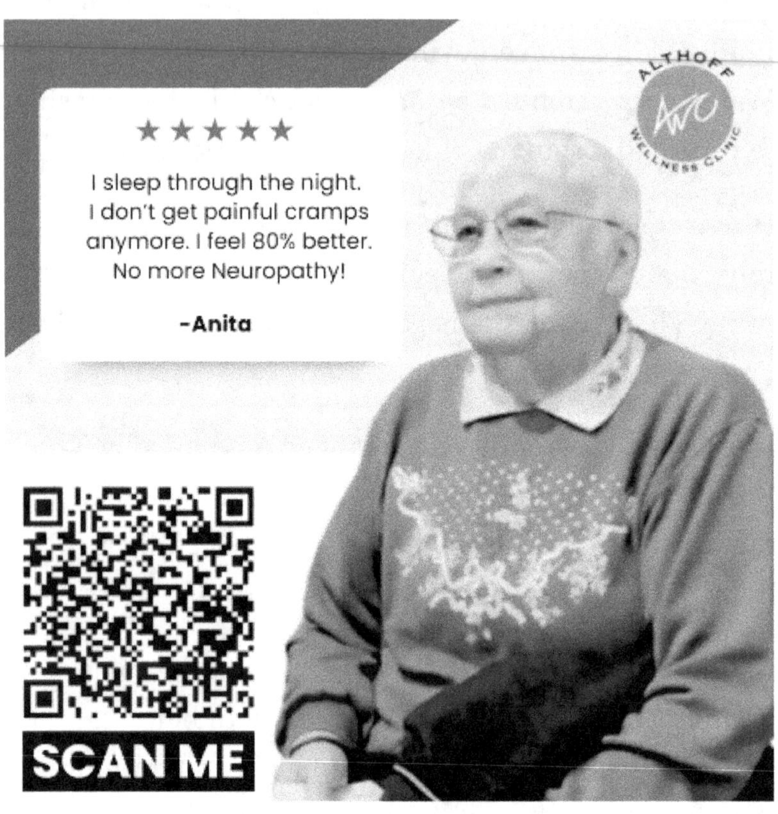

Unlock Your Path to Neuropathy Relief Now: Visit DrJillAlthoff.Com or Call (970) 579-7496 to Speak With Us Today!

Individual results may vary. Please review the disclaimer after the Table of Contents.

6

BLOOD SUGAR: THE HIDDEN ENEMY OF YOUR NERVES

I remember the weariness in Terri's voice when she first described her struggle with neuropathy. "My feet and legs ached constantly," she said, "especially at night. I couldn't sleep, and simple things like walking up the stairs felt impossible." Terri had tried everything to find relief, but the pain had begun to chip away at her spirit, making even a relaxing bath impossible.

Six weeks into the REPAIR program, I saw a remarkable change in Terri. Her eyes sparkled with newfound energy as she told me, "I can actually walk barefoot on my porch again! And I can finally sleep through the night!"

It's important to note that every patient's journey is unique. Terri's story is a powerful example of the potential benefits of this program, but individual results may vary. Witnessing Terri reclaim her daily joys is a constant reminder that neuropathy doesn't have to be a life sentence. By understanding the role of blood sugar in nerve health and embracing a holistic approach, we can empower our bodies to heal and thrive.

Think of your blood sugar like a mischievous gremlin riding a rollercoaster. One minute it's soaring with a sugary treat, the next it's plummeting into a dizzying drop after a missed meal. This erratic journey, unfortunately, is more than just a fleeting thrill ride; it can leave a trail of destruction in your body, especially for your delicate nerves.

This chapter is your guide to understanding the delicate dance between blood sugar and insulin, and their powerful role in preventing a sneaky culprit – peripheral neuropathy.

The Typical American Diet and Blood Sugar Imbalance

The American diet often prioritizes convenience and indulgence, significantly impacting your blood sugar levels and, subsequently, your nervous system. Let's explore how common dietary habits contribute to blood sugar imbalances and set the stage for peripheral neuropathy.

The Carb Rollercoaster: When you consume refined carbohydrates like white bread, sugary cereals, and pasta, your blood sugar spikes rapidly, giving you a quick burst of energy. However, it soon crashes, leaving you feeling tired and craving more sugar. This constant up-and-down cycle can lead to long-term damage.

Sugar Overload: Sugar is everywhere in the typical American diet – from soda to candy bars to flavored yogurts. Consuming too much sugar can cause your blood sugar to spike, forcing your body to produce more insulin to cope. Over time, this can lead to insulin resistance, a precursor to diabetes and neuropathy.

Processed foods, Inflammation and Oxidative Stress: Many processed foods are packed with unhealthy fats, sugars, and additives. The constant influx of sugar and processed foods leads to chronic inflammation and oxidative stress.. Chronic inflammation is harmful to your nerves. Think of inflammation as small fires burning inside your body, damaging your cells and your nerves. Imagine your body's cells as tiny engines. Processed foods clog these engines, making them work harder and eventually causing them to break down. Oxidative stress, on the other hand, is like rust that slowly deteriorates your nerves.

Sugar: The Addictive Substance

Sugar is not just a dietary concern; it's a powerful substance with addictive properties. Studies have shown that sugar can be more addictive than cocaine, activating the brain's reward centers and leading to cravings and overconsumption. This addiction exacerbates blood sugar imbalances, contributing to the development and progression of neuropathy.

The Insulin-Glucose Relationship: A Delicate Balance

Imagine glucose molecules as tiny particles moving through your bloodstream, with insulin acting as a key that unlocks cells to allow glucose in for energy. When you consume too much sugar, insulin struggles to keep up, and glucose lingers in the bloodstream, leading to high blood sugar levels.

Glucagon is like a backup system, releasing stored glucose from your liver when your blood sugar levels dip. This balance ensures a steady energy supply. But when insulin and glucagon are out of sync, your nerves can suffer.

High blood sugar is like sandpaper on delicate surfaces – it gradually wears down your nerves over time. If left unchecked, this imbalance can lead to neuropathy, characterized by a loss of sensation and balance.

Stages of Insulin Resistance: A Slow Decline

Insulin resistance is like a slow decline that starts subtly but can lead to severe complications. Understanding these stages can help you take action before it's too late.

A. Early Warning Signs: The Emergence of Insulin Resistance

- **Cellular Resistance:** Your cells become less responsive to insulin, causing sugar to linger in your bloodstream, leading to temporary spikes in blood sugar.
- **Elevated Post-Meal Sugar:** High blood sugar levels after meals indicate the beginning of insulin resistance. Although not yet dangerous, it signals potential trouble ahead.

B. Moderate Insulin Resistance: A Growing Neuropathy Risk

- **Impaired Glucose Tolerance:** Your body still tries to clear the sugar, but it takes longer. Prolonged high blood sugar levels can damage your nerves over time.

- **Abdominal Fat and Metabolic Syndrome:**
  Excess belly fat can worsen insulin resistance,
  creating a perfect storm for neuropathy.

C. Severe Insulin Resistance: The Tipping Point for Neuropathy

- **Chronic High Sugar:** Persistent high blood
  sugar levels directly damage nerves, leading to
  chronic hyperglycemia and neuropathy.
- **Beta-Cell Exhaustion:** Overworked pancreatic
  cells produce less insulin, leaving your nerves
  vulnerable to further damage.

Insulin Fatigue: When the System Wears Out

Think of your insulin as tireless workers trying to manage sugar levels. Over time, these workers can become exhausted, leading to insulin fatigue. Hyperinsulinemia, or high insulin levels, initially seems like a solution but eventually weakens your cells' response to insulin.

Prolonged high insulin levels damage your nerves, leading to tingling, numbness, and pain – early signs of neuropathy. If left unchecked, this can progress to type 2 diabetes, where your body fails to regulate blood sugar, causing further nerve damage.

Uncontrolled blood sugar is like a relentless storm, starving your nerves of oxygen and nutrients, damaging their protective sheaths, and disrupting their communication channels. This leads to various neuropathic complications, from pain and weakness to digestive issues and erectile dysfunction.

The New Fad: Semaglutides and Ozempic – A Double-Edged Sword

In recent years, medications like semaglutides (found in Ozempic) have gained popularity for managing blood sugar levels and aiding weight loss. While they can be effective tools, they also carry risks that could affect your delicate insulin balance and overall nerve health.

Mechanism of Action: Semaglutides mimic a hormone called GLP-1, which helps regulate insulin and blood sugar levels. They slow down digestion and reduce appetite, leading to better blood sugar control and weight loss.

Potential Downsides:

- **Gastrointestinal Issues:** These medications can cause nausea, vomiting, and diarrhea, which may lead to dehydration and electrolyte imbalances.

- **Pancreatitis Risk:** There is a potential risk of pancreatitis, an inflammation of the pancreas, which can affect insulin production and worsen blood sugar control.
- **Long-Term Effects:** The long-term effects on nerve health are not fully understood. While they may help manage blood sugar, relying solely on medications without lifestyle changes can mask underlying issues that need to be addressed for comprehensive nerve health.

Holistic Approach: While semaglutides can be part of a diabetes management plan, they should be used alongside dietary changes, regular exercise, and stress management to ensure a balanced approach to health.

Outsmarting Insulin Fatigue: Strategies for Nerve Health

To protect your nerves, it's crucial to prevent insulin fatigue and manage blood sugar levels effectively. Here are some strategies:

A. Dietary Delights: Fueling Your Cells the Right Way

- **Whole Foods:** Choose whole, unprocessed foods like fruits, vegetables, whole grains, and lean proteins. These release glucose slowly, keeping your energy levels steady.

- **Avoid Sugary and Processed Foods:** Ditch sugary treats and processed carbs that cause blood sugar spikes.

B. Beyond the Plate: Lifestyle Changes for Nerve Health

- **Regular Exercise:** Physical activity improves insulin sensitivity, helping your cells use glucose more efficiently.
- **Stress Management:** Chronic stress disrupts hormonal balance. Practice meditation or yoga to reduce stress and protect your nerves.

C. Functional Medicine: Digging Deeper for Root Causes

- **Identify Hidden Issues:** Functional medicine addresses the root causes of neuropathy risk, such as food intolerances, nutrient deficiencies, and gut imbalances.

D. Your Personalized Plan: Embracing Individuality

- **Individualized Care:** Work with a holistic healthcare professional to create a personalized plan for optimal blood sugar control and nerve protection.

Remember, you have the power to rewrite the narrative of your health. By making smart dietary choices, staying active, managing stress, and seeking personalized care, you can live a life free from the limitations of neuropathy.

ACTION STEP: Check Your Blood Sugar Levels

See if your blood sugar levels are higher than normal. If they are, getting them under control is crucial for reversing neuropathy symptoms. Testing your fasting blood glucose and HbA1c is important. Although we don't typically take blood in our office, we still recommend you get these tests done.

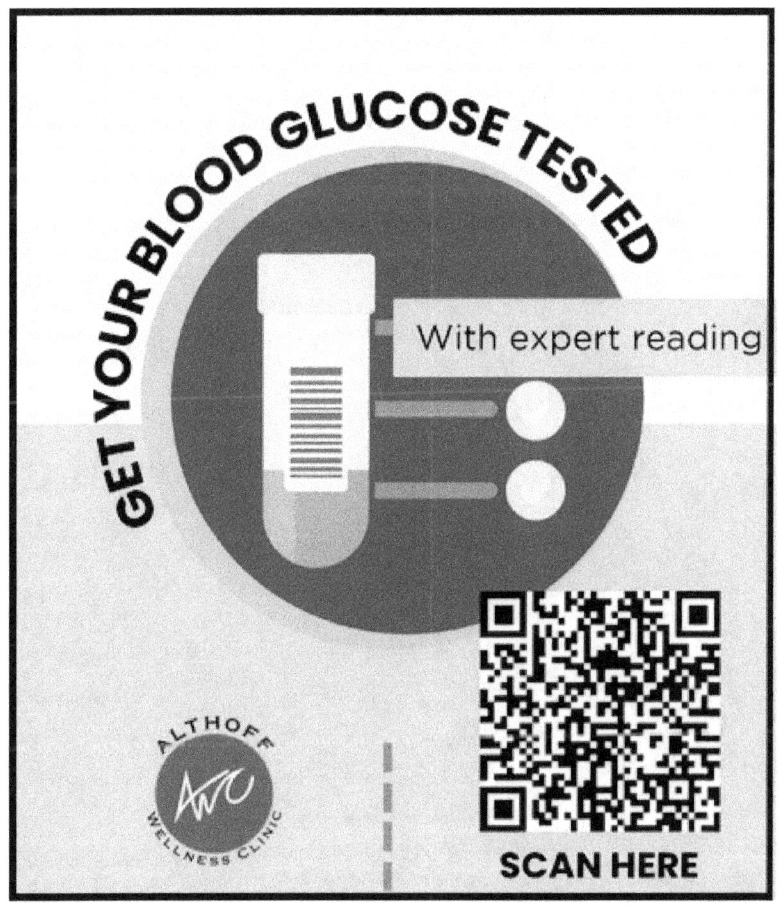

Unlock Your Path to Neuropathy Relief Now: Visit DrJillAlthoff.Com or Call (970) 579-7496 to Speak With Us Today!

Individual results may vary. Please review the disclaimer after the Table of Contents.

7

FUELING YOUR NERVES: THE POWER OF DIET AND EXERCISE

Ah, food! It's not just fuel for our bodies but a powerful tool in our neuropathy toolbox. Think of your nerves like delicate vines and your diet like the rich, nourishing soil they need to thrive. The right nutrients can rebuild and strengthen those pathways, pushing back against the tide of tingling, numbness, and pain.

Diet and Neuropathy: What to Eat and What to Avoid

Eating a balanced and nutritious diet is crucial for overall health and well-being, and it is especially important for individuals with neuropathy. Nutrient deficiencies, such as vitamin B12 deficiency, can worsen

81

neuropathy symptoms and slow down the healing process.

A balanced and nutritious diet should include a variety of whole foods, such as fruits, vegetables, whole grains, lean proteins, and healthy fats. These foods provide essential nutrients like vitamins, minerals, antioxidants, and omega-3 fatty acids, which support nerve health and function.

Foods That Can Impact Nerve Function

Certain foods and nutrients can impact nerve function positively or negatively. Here are some examples:

- **Antioxidants:** These nutrients protect the nerves from oxidative stress, which can damage nerve cells. Antioxidant-rich foods include berries, leafy greens, nuts, and seeds.
- **Omega-3 Fatty Acids:** These healthy fats support nerve function and reduce inflammation. Good sources of omega-3s include fatty fish, flaxseeds, and chia seeds.
- **Vitamin B12:** This vitamin is essential for nerve health and function. It can be found in animal products like meat, fish, and dairy.
- **High-Sugar Foods:** Foods high in sugar can cause blood sugar spikes and worsen

neuropathy symptoms. Examples include candy, soda, and baked goods.

- **Processed and Fried Foods:** These foods are often high in unhealthy fats and can worsen inflammation, which can worsen neuropathy symptoms. Examples include fast food, frozen meals, and snack foods.

Foods to Eat for Neuropathy

Let's discuss nutrient-dense foods that can support nerve health and the specific nutrients that are important for neuropathy management.

Some of the best foods for neuropathy are:

- **Fruits:** Rich in antioxidants, vitamins, minerals, and fiber. They help protect the nerves from oxidative stress, support blood sugar regulation, and promote gut health. Some of the best fruits for neuropathy are berries, melons, apples, and pears.
- **Vegetables:** High in antioxidants, vitamins, minerals, and fiber. They help reduce inflammation, improve nerve blood flow, and prevent constipation. Additionally, vegetables can help create a more basic pH level in the body, which promotes healing. Some of the

best vegetables for neuropathy are leafy greens (such as spinach), broccoli (which contains vitamin K), carrots (which contain beta-carotene), and sweet potatoes (which contain vitamin A).

- **Whole Grains:** Provide complex carbohydrates that give energy to the nerves. They also contain fiber that helps lower cholesterol and regulate blood sugar levels. Some of the best whole grains for neuropathy are oats (which contain beta-glucan), brown rice (which contains magnesium), quinoa (which contains iron), and barley (which contains selenium).

- **Lean Proteins:** Provide amino acids essential for building new nerve cells and repairing damaged ones. They also help maintain muscle mass and prevent weight loss. Some of the best lean proteins for neuropathy are chicken breast (which contains niacin), fish (which contains omega-3 fatty acids), eggs (which contain choline), and tofu (which contains calcium).

- **Healthy Fats:** Provide essential fatty acids that support nerve function and reduce inflammation. They also help lower blood pressure and cholesterol levels, improving blood circulation to the nerves. Some of the best healthy fats for neuropathy are olive oil (which contains oleic acid), avocado (which contains monounsaturated fat), nuts (which contain vitamin E), and seeds (which contain alpha-linolenic acid).

Methylated vs. Non-Methylated B Vitamins

When it comes to B vitamins, especially B12 and folate, the form you take can make a significant difference in how well your body utilizes these nutrients. This is particularly important for individuals with neuropathy.

- **Methylated B Vitamins:** Methylated vitamins are in their active form, meaning your body can use them directly without needing to convert them. This is crucial for people who have genetic mutations in the MTHFR gene, which affects the body's ability to methylate B vitamins. Methylated forms include methylcobalamin (B12) and methylfolate (folic acid). These forms are often better absorbed and utilized by the body, providing more immediate benefits for nerve health.

- **Non-Methylated B Vitamins:** These are the standard forms of B vitamins found in most supplements, such as cyanocobalamin (B12) and folic acid. These forms need to be converted into their active forms in the body. While some people can effectively use non-methylated forms, others may have difficulty due to genetic mutations or metabolic impairments. Additionally, cyanocobalamin, a common form of B12, is attached to a cyanide molecule, which is a toxin. Although the amount of cyanide is small, it's generally safer to choose methylcobalamin for better absorption and fewer risks.

Moving Towards Healing: Physical Therapy and Exercise in Neuropathy Management

Forget the dusty image of physical therapy filled with rigid stretches and boring machines. It's time to reimagine it as a dance party for your nerves, a celebration of movement, and a powerful tool in your neuropathy toolbox!

Physical activity may not cure neuropathy, but it can be the key to unlocking a life filled with more mobility, less pain, and a whole lot of fun. Here are just some of the other benefits of exercise for neuropathy:

- **Increasing Blood Flow:** Exercise helps increase blood flow to the nerves by dilating the blood vessels, which helps reduce nerve damage and pain.

- **Increasing Muscle Strength:** Exercise helps build muscle mass by stimulating the nerve endings in the muscles. This can help improve nerve function and prevent muscle atrophy.
- **Improving Balance:** Exercise helps improve balance by challenging your sensory system helping prevent falls and injuries.
- **Reducing Stress:** Exercise helps release endorphins, which are natural painkillers and mood enhancers, which can help reduce stress and anxiety.

So, grab your sneakers, ditch the doubt, and let's explore some of the best exercises for neuropathy:

Aerobic Exercises: These are exercises that raise your heart rate and breathing rate for a sustained period. They include walking, cycling, swimming, or dancing. Aerobic exercises can help improve your cardiovascular health and endurance.

Flexibility Training: These exercises stretch your muscles gently without causing pain or discomfort. They include yoga, Pilates, tai chi, or static stretching. Flexibility training can help improve your range of motion and prevent stiffness.

Balance and Strengthening Exercises for Neuropathy

Incorporating balance and strengthening exercises into your routine can significantly enhance your stability, muscle strength, and overall well-being. These exercises help prevent falls, stimulate nerve function, improve coordination, and prevent muscle atrophy. Here are some effective exercises you can do:

Balance and Strengthening Exercises

1. **Leg Raises:** Stand behind a chair and hold onto the back for support. Slowly lift one leg straight back without bending your knee or pointing your toes. Hold for a few seconds, then lower it back down. Repeat 10 to 15 times on each leg.
2. **Calf Raises:** Stand with your feet shoulder-width apart and hold onto a wall or chair for support. Lift your heels off the ground as high as you can, then slowly lower them back down. Repeat 10 to 15 times.
3. **Side Leg Raises:** Stand next to a wall or chair for support. Slowly lift one leg out to the side without tilting your body. Hold for a few seconds, then lower it back down. Repeat 10 to 15 times on each leg.

4. **Standing on One Leg:** Stand near a wall or chair for support. Lift one foot off the ground and balance on the other leg. Try to hold the position for 10 to 15 seconds, then switch legs. For an added challenge, try closing your eyes while balancing, but ensure you are in a safe environment where you can easily brace yourself if needed.

5. **Walking Heel to Toe:** Walk in a straight line, placing one foot directly in front of the other as if walking on a balance beam. Do this in a hallway so you can use the walls for support if needed. Repeat this for 10 to 15 steps.

6. **Toe Yoga:** While sitting or standing, try to raise your big toe while keeping all other toes on the ground. Then push the big toe down and raise all the other toes up. You may use your hands to help to start with. Repeat this 10 to 15 times.

7. **Toe Curls:** Sit on a chair with your feet flat on the floor. Curl your toes up as high as you can, then relax them. Repeat this 10 to 15 times.

8. **Heel Raises:** Stand with your feet shoulder-width apart and hold onto a wall or a chair for balance. Lift your heels off the ground as high as you can, then lower them slowly. Repeat this 10 to 15 times.

9. **Ankle Circles:** Sit on a chair with your feet flat on the floor. Rotate your ankles clockwise and counterclockwise for 10 seconds in each direction.

10. **Resistance Band Exercises:** Attach one end of the band to a fixed object at chest or waist level. Hold the other end of the band in one hand and perform various movements with that arm, such as bending it at the elbow or shoulder or extending it straight out or across your body. Repeat with the other arm.

Incorporating these balance and strengthening exercises into your daily routine can help improve your stability, muscle strength, and overall well-being. Always remember to consult with a healthcare professional before starting any new exercise program, especially if you have existing health conditions or concerns. By dedicating time to these exercises, you can significantly enhance your quality of life and manage neuropathy more effectively.

The Role of Stress Management

Stress management is a vital part of neuropathy relief. Stress can worsen your nerve pain, inflammation, and blood sugar levels, further damaging your nerves and organs. Stress can also affect your mood, sleep, appetite, and immune system, making you more vulnerable to infections and complications.

So, it's important to learn how to cope with stress in healthy ways and reduce its negative impact on your neuropathy condition. Here are some of the strategies that can help you manage stress and improve your neuropathy relief:

- **Cognitive-Behavioral Therapy (CBT):** This type of psychotherapy helps you identify and challenge negative thoughts and beliefs that cause or worsen your stress. CBT teaches you coping skills and relaxation techniques to deal with stressful situations and emotions. CBT has been shown to be effective in reducing neuropathic pain.
- **Mindfulness Meditation:** This practice involves paying attention to the present moment with curiosity and openness. Mindfulness meditation can help you reduce stress by lowering your blood pressure, heart rate, and cortisol levels. It can also help you increase awareness of your sensations, emotions, and thoughts without judging or reacting to them.

- **Yoga:** This form of physical exercise combines breathing, movement, and meditation. Yoga can help you reduce stress by improving your flexibility, strength, balance, and posture. It can also help you calm your mind and body by releasing endorphins, which are natural painkillers and mood enhancers.

- **Acupuncture:** This traditional Chinese medicine technique involves inserting thin needles into specific points on the body to stimulate the flow of energy or qi. Acupuncture can help you reduce stress by balancing your hormones, nerves, muscles, and organs. It can also help you relieve pain by blocking pain signals from reaching the brain.

- **Herbal Remedies:** Natural substances used for centuries to treat various health conditions. Some herbs that may help with neuropathy are ginkgo biloba, turmeric, ginger, chamomile, lavender, valerian root, passionflower, kava kava, St. John's wort, omega-3 fatty acids, and vitamin B12. Before taking any of these herbs, consult your doctor, as some may interact with your medications or have side effects. Follow the recommended dosage and instructions for each herb and monitor your symptoms and reactions.

Real-Life Transformations: The Power of Diet and Exercise in Action

We've explored the powerful impact of nutrition and movement on your nerve health. But let's move beyond the science and hear from someone who's experienced these benefits firsthand.

Meet Ray. Six months ago, Ray came to Althoff Wellness Clinic PC, seeking relief from the relentless grip of neuropathy. He was plagued by burning pain and tingling in his feet, especially at night. "It got so bad," Ray shares, "I'd resort to putting ice packs in my bed just to find some relief." These nighttime struggles disrupted his sleep, leaving him fatigued and dragging throughout the day. Even the simplest tasks, like walking, became a challenge. "If I looked up while walking," he recalls, "I'd swerve, like I'd been drinking or something. My balance was completely off."

Ray also experienced what he calls "ghost pains," sharp, shooting sensations that seemed to come out of nowhere, even while he was driving. These unpredictable pains, along with the constant burning and tingling, made him feel trapped in a cycle of discomfort with no escape. He had tried various treatments with little success, leading him to believe that neuropathy was something he'd simply have to learn to live with.

Then Ray discovered the REPAIR program. Along with the targeted therapies, a key component of his journey involved embracing the principles of nerve-nourishing nutrition and gentle movement. Ray committed to making gradual yet significant changes to his diet and daily routine. He swapped sugary snacks for vibrant vegetables and fiber-rich grains, providing his nerves with the steady fuel they craved. He incorporated gentle exercises into his day, improving circulation and boosting his overall well-being.

Six months later, Ray's story is one of hope and transformation. "The burning pain is significantly less," he says, a smile lighting up his face. "I'm sleeping better, and walking feels so much easier. The ghost pains are far less frequent too. There are still things to work on, but it's incredible how much things have changed."

While everyone's journey with neuropathy is unique, Ray's story highlights the profound impact of diet and exercise on nerve health, especially when combined with other elements of the REPAIR program. His story is a testament to the power of embracing a holistic approach, one that nourishes your body, calms inflammation, and awakens your inner healing mechanisms, paving the way for a life free from the grip of neuropathy.

ACTION STEP: Scan the code below to download our 25 Anti-Inflammatory Recipes Guide.

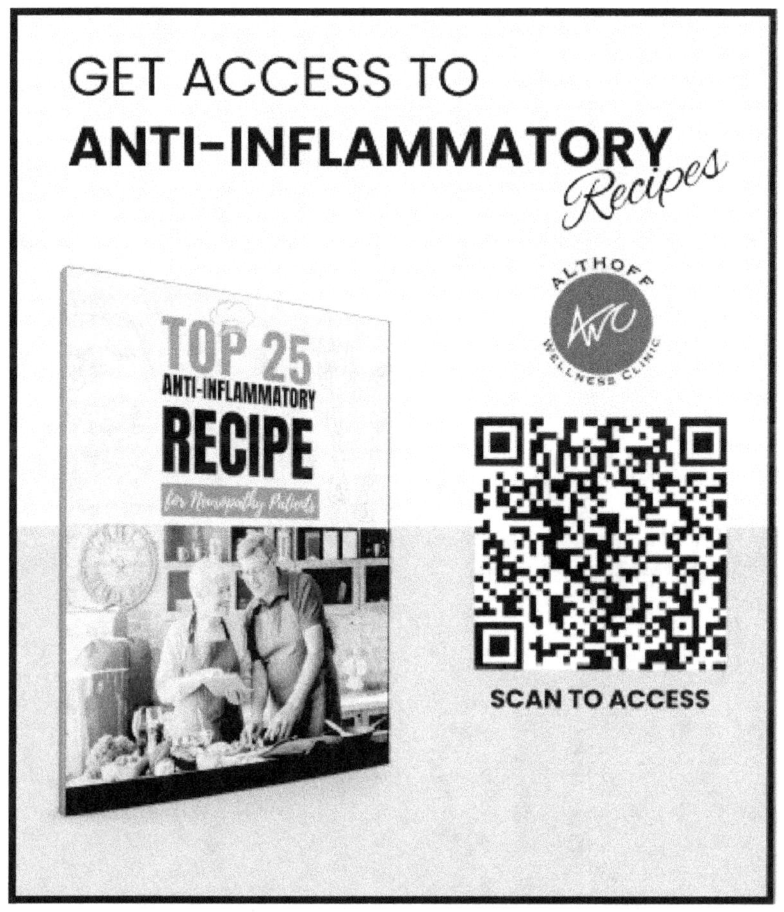

Unlock Your Path to Neuropathy Relief Now: Visit DrJillAlthoff.Com or Call (970) 579-7496 to Speak With Us Today!

Individual results may vary. Please review the disclaimer after the Table of Contents.

8

YOUR NERVOUS SYSTEM UNDER ATTACK: THE MECHANISMS OF NEUROPATHY

There's a palpable sense of relief when a patient regains their footing, literally and metaphorically. I recall the day Hank walked into my office, a hesitant smile on his face. "I used to feel like my legs would just go to sleep during the day," he confessed, "like they were made of wood." Neuropathy had robbed him of the simple joy of feeling the ground beneath his feet, making every step uncertain.

But after a few months in the REPAIR program, a noticeable change occurred. Hank's stride was more confident, his smile brighter. He shared how the numbness was receding, how he was regaining sensation. He was even able to stand on one leg during our balance exercises—a feat that had seemed impossible just weeks earlier. It's moments like these that fuel my passion for helping people like Hank reconnect with their bodies and reclaim their lives from the grip of neuropathy.

Success with this program is not guaranteed for everyone. However, it's inspiring to see how Hank has made such progress. If you or someone you love is struggling with peripheral neuropathy, contact us today and find out how we can help you.

Imagine your body as a bustling city, with your nervous system as the intricate network of highways connecting everything. This system transmits a constant stream of information, controlling everything from how you walk and talk to the digestion of your food and the steady beat of your heart. Your nerves are the tireless messengers, keeping the city running smoothly.

Unfortunately, neuropathy disrupts this finely tuned communication network. Think of it like worn-out cables causing static on the line. Those once-clear signals your nerves send get garbled, leading to the burning, tingling, or numbness you experience in your feet, legs, or hands. But the impact of neuropathy goes beyond these sensations.

Disrupted nerve signals can affect your balance, making everyday activities like walking a challenge. They can interfere with digestion, causing bloating or other digestive issues. Even your sleep can suffer as those misfiring signals keep you up at night, making it difficult to get the rest you need.

The good news? Your body has a remarkable ability to heal itself, and that extends to your nervous system. While neuropathy can feel overwhelming, the REPAIR approach focuses on harnessing this natural healing potential. We'll create an environment where damaged nerves can begin to regenerate, and your body can reclaim its optimal function. Let's go on this journey together and get your body's information highway humming smoothly once again.

Understanding Your Nervous System: Friend or Foe in Neuropathy?

Let's explore the intricate world of your nervous system and see how neuropathy disrupts its delicate dance. Imagine it as a two-part system, working in beautiful harmony:

- **Central Nervous System (CNS):** This is your body's mission control – the brain and spinal cord. They're the masterminds, processing information, generating thoughts and emotions, and sending instructions to the rest of your body like a general to its troops.

- **Peripheral Nervous System (PNS):** Picture the PNS as a vast communication network branching out from your spinal cord. Think of countless phone lines connecting your CNS to every nook and cranny – your organs, muscles, and even your skin. This network is responsible for relaying sensations (like touch and temperature), controlling movement, and even managing some automatic functions like your heart rate. It's here, in this peripheral system, where neuropathy primarily wreaks havoc.

Now, let's zoom in on a single nerve, the workhorse of the PNS. Imagine a tiny cable – the core wire carrying the message is called the axon. Wrapped around this axon is a fatty layer called the myelin sheath. Think of it like the insulating coat on an electrical wire, protecting the signal it carries.

When neuropathy strikes, it can damage both the axon and the myelin sheath. Damaged insulation, like faulty wiring, scrambles the message, leading to pain. Or, if the "wire" itself is broken, it can cause numbness. These injured nerves are causing frustrating neuropathy symptoms that people experience.

By understanding this communication breakdown, we can develop strategies to repair the damage and restore harmony to your nervous system. The REPAIR program will be your guide, helping you create an environment where your nerves can heal and function optimally once again.

The Plot Twist: How Nerves Get Hijacked in Neuropathy

Our amazing nervous system, usually a marvel of communication, can sometimes take a wrong turn. This detour is what we call neuropathy, and it can manifest in a few different ways:

- **Peripheral Neuropathy:** This is our area of focus. It's when the nerves in your extremities – feet, hands, legs, and sometimes arms – malfunction. This is the culprit behind the uncomfortable tingling, burning, and numbness you might experience.
- **Autonomic Neuropathy:** This less common type disrupts the nerves that control your body's "automatic" functions, like digestion, heart rate, and blood pressure. While less frequent, it's important to be aware of it.

So, what triggers this nerve hijacking? It's rarely a single villain. Instead, a combination of factors often team up to create a domino effect of damage. Let's explore some of the main culprits:

- **Blood Sugar Rollercoaster:** Unstable blood sugar levels wreak havoc on your entire body, including your nerves. When sugar levels spike and crash, it throws everything off balance.
- **Chronic Inflammation:** Imagine a constant low-grade fire burning throughout your body. This inflammation can wreak havoc on delicate nerves, making them particularly vulnerable.
- **Nutritional Shortfalls:** Nerves, like high-performance athletes, need specific vitamins and minerals to function optimally and repair themselves. When your diet lacks these essential nutrients, your nerve health suffers.
- **Underlying Medical Conditions:** Diabetes is the most well-known risk factor, but neuropathy can also be a sidekick to conditions like autoimmune disorders, thyroid problems, and even past infections or exposure to toxins.

Here's the crucial point: To truly conquer neuropathy, we need to be detectives, not just symptom suppressors. We need to delve deeper, identify the root causes of the disruption, and address these directly. The REPAIR program will be your partner in this detective work, helping you uncover the culprit and create a personalized plan for optimal nerve health.

Unleashing Your Body's Inner Healer: The Power of Neuroplasticity

Here's the incredible truth: your body isn't a rigid machine; it's a dynamic force with an amazing capacity to heal itself, and that includes your nerves. This is where the fascinating concept of neuroplasticity comes in.

Think of your brain and nerves as a complex electrical grid. Neuroplasticity is the brain's remarkable ability to adapt, rewire, and form new connections – like rewiring a damaged circuit board. While it doesn't happen overnight, it's the cornerstone of true healing for neuropathy.

So, how do we tap into this natural superpower? Let's explore the tools:

- **Feeding Your Nerves:** Your nerves are like high-performance athletes – they crave specific nutrients to function optimally and repair themselves. B vitamins, magnesium, and other key nutrients act as building blocks for repair and shields against further damage. The REPAIR program will guide you on fortifying your diet with these essential nerve fuel sources.

- **Lifestyle as Medicine:** Simple, yet powerful, lifestyle adjustments play a crucial role. Getting restorative sleep, managing stress effectively, and engaging in the right types of movement all work together to reduce inflammation and create an environment conducive to nerve healing.

- **The REPAIR Advantage:** Our comprehensive approach goes beyond just support. The REPAIR therapies are specifically designed to directly stimulate nerve regeneration, increase blood flow to damaged areas, and calm the chronic "fire" of inflammation. Combined with targeted nutrition and those lifestyle shifts, this creates a powerful synergy for healing, accelerating your journey back to vibrant nerve health.

Remember, healing is a marathon, not a sprint. Consistency is key. By understanding and actively supporting your body's innate healing mechanisms, you unlock the potential for real, lasting improvement in your neuropathy. The REPAIR program will be your partner on this journey, empowering you to take charge of your health and reclaim the life you deserve.

Tapping into the Mind-Body Connection: Your Secret Weapon Against Neuropathy

Healing is often viewed as a purely physical process, but when it comes to neuropathy, we can't overlook the powerful mind-body connection. Here's why it matters:

Stress: The Silent Saboteur

Chronic stress throws your body into a constant state of "fight or flight." This stress response floods your system with hormones that worsen inflammation, ultimately amplifying your neuropathy symptoms. It also keeps your body focused on survival, making healing a secondary concern.

Stress Relief: The Healing Catalyst

Learning to manage stress isn't just about feeling better in the moment, it's about unlocking your body's natural healing potential. Here are some powerful tools to consider:

- **Mindfulness Practices:** Simple exercises like focusing on your breath for a few minutes can bring you into the present moment, calming a racing mind. Techniques like meditation can become a powerful ally in your fight against neuropathy.

- **Gentle Movement:** Yoga, Tai Chi, or even mindful walking are excellent ways to release tension and improve circulation, both of which can significantly benefit your nerves.
- **Guided Relaxation:** Many apps and audio recordings offer guided meditations, making it easier to shift into a more relaxed state.

The key is finding what resonates with you. Even dedicating 5-10 minutes daily to these practices can make a world of difference in managing your stress and supporting your body's natural healing mechanisms. The REPAIR program will provide you with additional resources and guidance to help you cultivate this mind-body connection and empower your healing journey.

Cultivating Your Inner Strength: The Power of a Positive Mindset

You might think a positive mindset is just sunshine and rainbows, but when it comes to neuropathy, it's a force multiplier for your healing journey. Here's why:

The Self-Fulfilling Prophecy

If you believe your neuropathy will only worsen and keep you trapped, those thoughts become a self-fulfilling prophecy, hindering progress. However, when you cultivate the belief that healing is possible, you're more likely to embrace the REPAIR program with enthusiasm and commitment.

Mind Over Matter

A positive mindset won't cure neuropathy overnight. But it's a powerful tool. It reduces stress (remember our stress enemy?), increases motivation to follow through with the REPAIR program, and empowers you to face challenges with greater resilience.

Hope as Fuel

The road to recovery can be long. But believing in your body's ability to heal and having faith in the REPAIR process can make all the difference. It fuels your commitment, even when progress feels slow. It's important to acknowledge challenges, but don't let fear or past disappointments steal your hope. Empower yourself by focusing on the potential for a brighter and healthier future.

You Are in Charge

By now, you've gained a deeper understanding of your amazing nervous system and how neuropathy disrupts its delicate dance. This knowledge is more than just facts; it's about empowerment. The more you understand, the clearer it becomes that you're not just a victim of this condition; you're an active participant in your healing journey.

REPAIR: Your Partner in Healing

The REPAIR program is designed as a collaborative effort. We acknowledge the complexity of neuropathy by addressing not just the physical damage, but also the mental, emotional, and lifestyle factors that significantly impact your overall nerve health.

Think of it like this: Your nerves are that intricate communication network. Althoff Wellness Clinic PC is the REPAIR technician that you call when you are having problems. We'll provide the tools to mend damaged "wires," improve signal quality, and even help your brain and body establish healthier communication patterns. This multi-faceted approach is what sets REPAIR apart, offering true holistic healing and the best chance of lasting relief from neuropathy.

So, let's cultivate a positive mindset together, because with the right tools and unwavering belief in your potential, you can overcome the challenges of neuropathy and reclaim your vibrant health. The REPAIR program is here to guide you every step of the way.

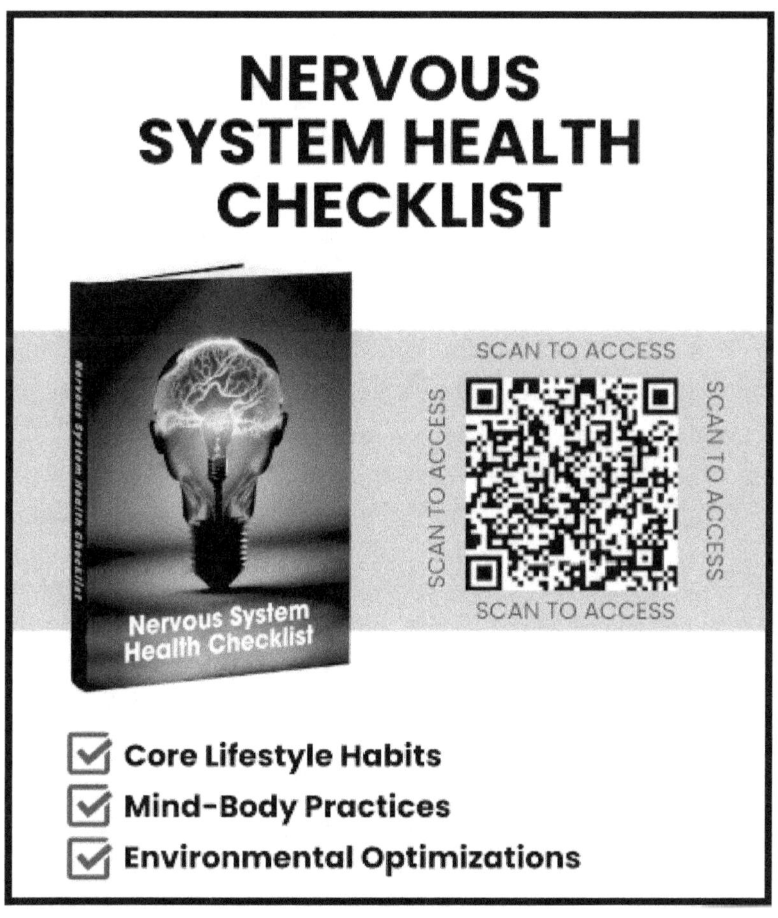

Unlock Your Path to Neuropathy Relief Now: Visit DrJillAlthoff.Com or Call (970) 579-7496 to Speak With Us Today!

Individual results may vary. Please review the disclaimer after the Table of Contents.

9

———

**TOXINS AND NEUROPATHY: A
HIDDEN RISK**

If you're battling neuropathy, it's crucial to understand the role toxins play in your condition. While statins are a well-known culprit, they're not the only toxic threat to your nerve health. Various toxins, including chemotherapy drugs, heavy metals, and certain environmental pollutants, can cause or worsen neuropathy. This chapter will delve into the different types of toxins that pose risks and offer guidance on how to protect yourself.

The Role of Toxins in Neuropathy

Toxicity-related peripheral neuropathy can result from exposure to various harmful substances. These toxins can damage nerves, leading to symptoms such as pain,

III

tingling, numbness, and weakness. Let's explore some common toxins that contribute to neuropathy:

1. **Chemotherapy Drugs.** Chemotherapy induced peripheral neuropathy (CIPN) is a significant side effect reported by many cancer patients. Chemotherapy drugs, particularly those used in high doses or on frequent treatment schedules, are notorious for causing neuropathy. These drugs target cancer cells but can also damage peripheral nerves, leading to debilitating symptoms.

2. **Heavy Metals.** Exposure to heavy metals like lead, mercury, and arsenic can result in neuropathy. These metals can accumulate in the body and disrupt nerve function. Industrial workers, those exposed to contaminated water, and individuals using certain traditional remedies are at higher risk. Knowledge is key. We encourage you to research anything you are putting into your body or activities that could be hazardous to your overall health. Investigate the pros and cons, potential side effects, or hazardous warnings to your health. Ask for a second opinion if you are ever in doubt, have additional questions, or simply don't feel like you are getting all the information you need.

3. **Environmental Pollutants.** Pesticides, solvents, and other environmental pollutants can also contribute to neuropathy. Long-term exposure to these substances, often found in agricultural and industrial settings, can damage nerves and lead to chronic pain and sensory issues.

Statins: A Double-Edged Sword

Statins are widely prescribed medications for lowering cholesterol. Let's dig a little deeper here. While these may seem like a straightforward solution for high cholesterol, the story for neuropathy patients is more complex.

Statins: Curbing Cholesterol Production

Imagine your liver as a factory churning out cholesterol. Statins act like production line supervisors, slowing down this process to bring down cholesterol levels. Sounds beneficial, right? Well, hold on...

The CoQ10 Conundrum

The plot thickens because your liver isn't just a cholesterol factory. It also manufactures CoQ10, a vital cellular fuel powering every cell in your body. Think of CoQ10 as the spark plugs in your car's engine. Here's the rub: statins can impede the CoQ10 production pathway. In other words, lowering cholesterol might come at the cost of depleted CoQ10 levels.

Why CoQ10 Matters for Your Nerves

Your nerves and muscles are particularly reliant on this fuel. When CoQ10 stores run low, it can lead to symptoms that mirror neuropathy – weakness, pain, and fatigue. This explains the concerning link between statin use and an increased risk of neuropathy or worsening existing symptoms.

Beyond Neuropathy: A Wider Web of Side Effects

Statins aren't without broader side effects. Muscle aches, difficulty concentrating (brain fog), blood sugar fluctuations, and even a potential rise in risk for Parkinson's or liver damage are all on the table. While some consider these side effects "mild," they can significantly impact your quality of life, especially when you're already managing neuropathy.

Understanding this potential downside of statins empowers you to ask informed questions and explore alternative approaches to managing your cholesterol and neuropathy. The REPAIR program will work with you to create a personalized plan that addresses both conditions without compromising your well-being.

Statins and Neuropathy: Navigating the Research Maze

Statins and neuropathy – the research paints a complex picture. Let's dig into the evidence and explore why this necessitates careful consideration when making treatment decisions.

Certain factors elevate your risk of statin-induced neuropathy:

- **Pre-existing Neuropathy or Diabetes:** If your nerves are already compromised, statins can further weaken them.
- **Age:** As we age, our bodies process medications less efficiently, increasing the likelihood of side effects.
- **Polypharmacy:** Taking multiple medications can create interactions, raising complication risks when combined with statins.
- **Vitamin D Deficiency:** Low Vitamin D levels may worsen the nerve-damaging effects of statins.

The Misdiagnosis Trap

Imagine this: you're taking a statin, and your neuropathy worsens – increased burning, weakness, and walking difficulties. Often, the assumption (even by some doctors) is that the neuropathy itself is simply progressing. This can lead to:

- **Escalating Statin Doses:** The thought process is, "Lower cholesterol is better, so let's increase the medication." Unfortunately, this can exacerbate side effects.
- **A Cocktail of Medications:** Doctors might prescribe additional medications to target nerve pain, overlooking the statin as a potential culprit.
- **Unnecessary Anxiety:** The belief that the condition is worsening can add mental and emotional stress to the physical challenges.

Here's the plot twist: some patients with statin-induced neuropathy experience initial improvement due to lowered cholesterol. This can create a false sense of security, masking the long-term nerve damage caused by the statin.

The key takeaway? Any change in your neuropathy symptoms (positive or negative) while taking statins warrants a thorough discussion with your doctor. Don't always assume these changes are simply the disease progressing.

Empowering Your Heart & Nerves: Natural Strategies for Optimal Health

There's fantastic news: safeguarding your heart doesn't have to rely solely on medications like statins. Natural approaches offer a powerful, multifaceted way to support your cardiovascular system and address the very issues that accelerate neuropathy.

Looking Beyond Cholesterol

Imagine inflammation as a relentless fire burning within your blood vessels. Over time, this fire damages the delicate lining, making it rough and sticky. This is where cholesterol steps in, potentially building up into dangerous plaques that can lead to heart attack or stroke. Statins address high cholesterol numbers, but they don't extinguish the underlying fire.

Oxidative Damage: The Silent Culprit

Another key player is oxidative damage. Think of all your cells, including those lining your blood vessels, as constantly producing "exhaust fumes" from their energy production processes. Antioxidants are your body's air filtration system, neutralizing those fumes. When chronic inflammation and an unhealthy lifestyle overload this system, it's like your blood vessels rusting from the inside out.

The Nerve Connection

Why is this relevant for neuropathy? Your nerves are hypersensitive to both inflammation and oxidative damage. The very things harming your heart are also contributing to the breakdown of your nerves. By addressing these root issues, you're not just protecting your heart – you're safeguarding your entire body, especially those vulnerable nerves.

Lifestyle as Your Medicine

Let's explore the power of lifestyle changes in protecting your heart and nerves. Prioritizing an anti-inflammatory diet is key. This means ditching processed foods and filling your plate with vibrant, whole foods. Think of all those colorful fruits and vegetables as an army of antioxidants, fighting free radicals and guarding your blood vessels and nerves. It's also crucial to choose foods that stabilize your blood sugar, as those spikes can cause widespread damage, particularly to sensitive nerves.

Don't underestimate the power of movement, even with neuropathy limitations. Find what works for you, whether it's short walks, chair-based exercises, or gentle water aerobics. Moving your body boosts circulation (essential for healing nerves) and helps your body combat chronic inflammation.

Finally, remember that stress management isn't a luxury, it's a necessity. When you're constantly in "fight or flight" mode, stress hormones wreak havoc on both your heart and nerves. Simple mindfulness practices, deep breathing exercises, or even taking a few minutes for a relaxing hobby can make a significant difference when done consistently.

Supplements: Targeted Support

While a healthy diet and lifestyle are foundational, targeted supplements can further enhance your heart and nerve protection. Omega-3 fatty acids, found in fish oil, are superstars at taming inflammation, benefiting both your blood vessels and those sensitive nerves.

Certain nutrients act like your body's internal blood sugar management team. Magnesium and alpha-lipoic acid are key players, helping to keep blood sugar levels steady and preventing those harmful spikes that contribute to neuropathy.

Lastly, antioxidants like resveratrol (found in grapes and red wine) and turmeric (the bright yellow spice) provide unique protective benefits for your heart and circulatory system, acting as a shield against oxidative damage.

Important Note: Remember, supplements are most effective when combined with healthy lifestyle changes.

Before adding any supplements, always consult with your doctor, especially if you take other medications. The REPAIR program can help you navigate these lifestyle changes and create a personalized plan to optimize your heart health and nerve function.

You in Charge: Making Informed Decisions About Statins and Your Nerves

This chapter isn't about demonizing statins but about empowering you with knowledge to make the best choices for your unique health situation. Whether you're currently taking statins or considering them, here's a roadmap to navigate this conversation:

Collaboration is Key: If you're already on statins, remember, abruptly stopping can be risky. There's a potential for cholesterol rebound. Working with your doctor is essential for a safe transition, which might involve gradually tapering off the medication or exploring alternative approaches.

Empowering Questions: Your next doctor's appointment shouldn't be a passive one. Here are some questions to champion your own health:

- "What are my specific heart disease risks, and how exactly does this statin medication help lower them?"

- "Are there lifestyle changes I can make that could potentially reduce my reliance on medication?"
- "If I experience any new muscle weakness, pain, or changes in thinking, should I report them immediately?"
- "Can we discuss alternative approaches to managing cholesterol besides statins, and weigh the pros and cons of each?"

The REPAIR Advantage: A Multifaceted Approach

Even when statins are deemed necessary, the REPAIR approach remains crucial. By addressing underlying causes like inflammation and blood sugar imbalances, you're protecting both your heart and nerves while potentially minimizing the long-term risks associated with statin use. It's about crafting a personalized plan, not a one-size-fits-all solution.

Throughout this chapter, we've explored how statins work, their potential downsides, and the power of natural approaches that nourish your entire body. This knowledge isn't meant to scare you but to empower you. By understanding your medications, you transform from a passive recipient of care into an active participant in your health journey.

Remember, the ultimate goal isn't just lowering a number on a lab test. True health means thriving nerves, a strong heart, and a life where medications are tools to support your well-being, not a life sentence. Striking a balance between heart health and nerve protection is absolutely achievable. This often involves a combination of smart lifestyle changes, targeted supplements, and carefully considered medications when truly necessary. The REPAIR program can guide you through this process, helping you create a personalized plan to achieve optimal health and reclaim your quality of life.

Finding Relief After Statins: Glen's Journey to Reclaimed Mobility

Glen, an avid hiker, first sought help at Althoff Wellness Clinic PC because of a growing concern: neuropathy was slowly robbing him of his ability to enjoy his favorite pastime. "My feet were getting progressively numb," Glen recalls. "I could barely feel my toes, and the numbness was starting to creep up my legs. I was worried about what this meant for my future."

His neuropathy made walking incredibly painful, especially after a hike. "I remember going on three-to-five-mile hikes with my son," Glen shares, "and by the time we got back, my feet would be absolutely killing me. It was so bad that I would wonder if I could even finish the hike. I knew I had to do something."

After undergoing extensive testing at Althoff Wellness Clinic PC, we discovered a possible culprit contributing to Glen's neuropathy: statins. While effective in managing his cholesterol, the statins seemed to be negatively impacting his nerve health.

Glen began a personalized treatment program incorporating the REPAIR principles, which included addressing the potential side effects of statins. "The treatment wasn't a quick fix," Glen explains, "It took time and dedication. But gradually, I started to feel the numbness receding. I could actually feel hot and cold in my feet again! And the pain after a hike was dramatically reduced."

A year later, Glen is back on the trails, enjoying his hikes with newfound confidence. "My feet can still get sore after a long hike," Glen admits, "but it's nothing like before. It's more like normal muscle soreness. I feel like I'm finally regaining control over my body."

Success with this program is not guaranteed for everyone. However, Glen's story highlights the critical need to be aware of the potential side effects of statins, especially for those experiencing neuropathy symptoms. It underscores the importance of seeking personalized care that addresses all aspects of your health, not just managing cholesterol. Glen's journey is a testament to the power of natural, holistic therapies in restoring nerve function and reclaiming the joy of movement, even after statin use.

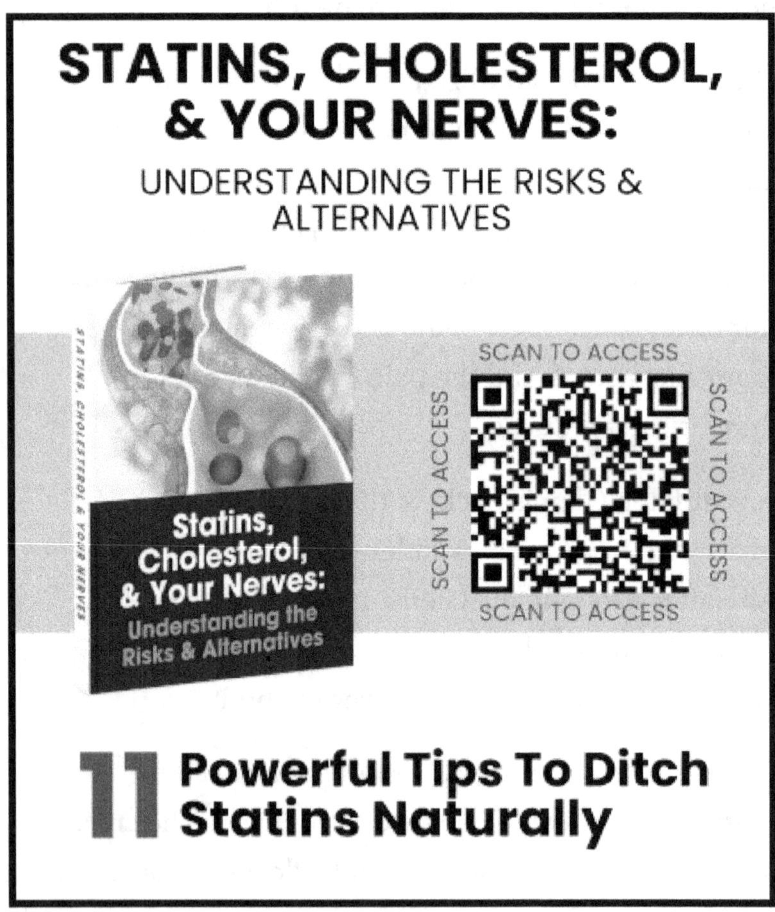

Unlock Your Path to Neuropathy Relief Now: Visit DrJillAlthoff.Com or Call (970) 579-7496 to Speak With Us Today!

125

Individual results may vary. Please review the disclaimer after the Table of Contents.

10

INFLAMMATION, LEAKY GUT, AND YOUR NERVES: THE GLUTEN CONNECTION

Let's delve into the world of gluten, that ever-present protein lurking in many of our favorite foods. If you're battling neuropathy, understanding gluten's potential impact on your health could be a turning point.

Consider how our diets have drastically changed. Gone are the days of gluten simply being in bread. It's snuck into processed foods, sauces, and even medications, leading to constant exposure – especially for those with hidden sensitivities.

The debate surrounding gluten is real. Some doctors dismiss it as a passing fad, while others are witnessing a clear link between gluten and various health issues, including neuropathy. The truth is, it likely doesn't affect everyone equally. But the growing body of research suggesting a connection between gluten and nerve damage is undeniable.

Here's the key takeaway: celiac disease isn't the only concern. Gluten sensitivity exists on a spectrum. Even milder forms can trigger significant inflammation throughout your body, and unfortunately, your nerves are susceptible to this inflammatory response.

Gluten: Friend or Foe for Your Nerves?

Let's break down the science behind gluten and why it can become a problem for some people with neuropathy.

Gluten itself isn't inherently bad. It's a protein found in wheat, rye, and barley. The issue arises from our modern diet's overabundance of gluten and how some bodies react to this constant bombardment.

The Problem with Gluten Sensitivity: In people with gluten sensitivity, their bodies struggle to properly digest this protein. Imagine tiny velcro hooks lining their gut. Gluten acts like these hooks, clinging to and irritating the delicate intestinal lining. This creates "leaky gut," where undigested food particles, toxins, and bacteria seep into the bloodstream.

Why Leaky Gut Matters for Nerves: Leaky gut triggers a full-blown inflammatory response throughout your body. Remember, inflammation is a major culprit in neuropathy.

Mistaken Identity: A Deceptive Disguise: Think of your immune system as a highly trained security team. They are constantly on the lookout for invaders like viruses and bacteria, which they identify based on specific "mugshots" (proteins or antigens). Sometimes, proteins from pathogens (like viruses or bacteria) share structural similarities with proteins found in your body's own cells. This resemblance can cause the immune system to mistake your own cells for invaders. When gluten triggers inflammation, it can lead the immune system to attack your nerve cells by mistake, causing further damage and worsening neuropathy symptoms.

The Gluten-Neuropathy Connection: Inflammation and Nerve Damage

We've explored how gluten sensitivity can trigger widespread inflammation throughout your body. But how does this translate to your experience with neuropathy?

Inflammation: The Silent Saboteur Neuropathy is essentially nerve damage that disrupts the communication between your nerves and your brain.

Inflammation throws a wrench into this delicate system in two ways:

- **Direct Irritation:** Inflammation acts like an irritant to your nerves, causing them to misfire and send those painful tingling, burning, or numbness sensations.
- **Healing Roadblock:** Inflammation also hinders the body's natural repair mechanisms, making it harder for damaged nerves to heal themselves.

Symptoms That Might Point to Gluten Sensitivity
Several symptoms often overlap with gluten sensitivity, making it a potential culprit worth exploring:

- **Digestive Distress:** Bloating, gas, diarrhea, or constipation often manifest as the first signs of gluten sensitivity in your gut.
- **Brain Fog:** Difficulty concentrating, fatigue, and mood swings can be linked to inflammation originating in the gut.
- **Aches and Pains:** Unexplained muscle or joint pain could be a sign of systemic inflammation triggered by gluten.
- **Skin Concerns:** Eczema, rashes, and other skin

problems often have a connection to gut-related inflammation.

Individual Responses: A Spectrum of Improvement

It's important to remember that responses to a gluten-free diet can vary greatly. For some people, eliminating gluten can lead to dramatic improvements in their neuropathy symptoms. For others, the effects may be more subtle but still a significant piece of the healing puzzle.

The key takeaway? Exploring potential triggers like gluten and managing inflammation are crucial steps on your journey to neuropathy repair. If you suspect gluten might be playing a role in your neuropathy, consulting with a healthcare professional can help you determine if a gluten-free trial might be right for you.

Unveiling Gluten's Role: Testing and Beyond

Unfortunately, figuring out if gluten is a culprit in your neuropathy isn't always a simple blood test. Let's explore why that is and delve into more reliable ways to find your answer.

The Limitations of Celiac Testing Standard celiac tests focus on identifying only a few specific types of antibodies. While a positive test strongly indicates celiac disease, a negative one isn't always definitive.

Here's the catch: Your immune system might be reacting to gluten in other ways. Maybe it involves different antibodies or an inflammatory response that doesn't show up on the standard panel. This means you could still be negatively affected by gluten despite a "normal" test result.

The bottom line? Your body's response to gluten can be more nuanced than a single test can always capture. This is why an elimination diet, where you become your own detective, can be a more reliable tool.

The Elimination Diet: Your Personal Investigation
This approach involves completely removing gluten from your diet for at least 3-4 weeks, followed by a reintroduction phase. While seemingly straightforward, there are key details for accurate results:

- **Strict Elimination:** Gluten can lurk in unexpected places. Meticulous label reading is essential.
- **Track Your Progress:** Monitor not just your neuropathy symptoms, but also digestion, energy levels, and any other improvements you might experience.
- **Mindful Reintroduction:** Pay close attention to how you feel after reintroducing gluten. A

significant increase in symptoms is your answer.

Going Gluten-Free: Benefits and Challenges

While removing gluten can be incredibly beneficial, it's important to be aware of the following:

Nutritional Gaps: Whole grains offer valuable nutrients like fiber, iron, and B vitamins. Don't fall into the trap of simply replacing gluten-containing foods with processed gluten-free alternatives. Focus on incorporating naturally gluten-free whole foods like quinoa, buckwheat, brown rice, legumes, and a rainbow of fruits and vegetables. This ensures your body gets the essential nutrients it needs for nerve repair.

Social Considerations: Eating out or at friends' houses requires extra planning. Research menus beforehand, possibly bring your own safe options, and advocate for yourself when necessary. Finding a supportive community, whether online or in-person, can be invaluable as you navigate this change.

Not a Standalone Solution: While gluten can be a major trigger for some, it's rarely the sole culprit. Neuropathy is complex. Optimizing blood sugar regulation, addressing other inflammatory factors, and potentially incorporating targeted therapies like those in the REPAIR program may still be necessary for optimal healing.

Think of going gluten-free as clearing a major roadblock on your path to recovery. It creates a more favorable environment for your body – and the REPAIR approach – to work its magic and promote nerve healing!

Finding Relief by Breaking the Chains: Patty's Journey Beyond Gluten

Patty came to Althoff Wellness Clinic PC seeking relief from a frustrating combination of symptoms. "It was a struggle just to get through the day," Patty recalls. "My feet and legs ached constantly, and it was especially bad at night. I couldn't sleep, and going up and down stairs was incredibly painful." The pain limited Patty's ability to travel and enjoy time with her family. "My family was constantly worried about me," she shares, "because they could see how much I was struggling."

Patty had tried everything to ease her discomfort, from changing her shoes multiple times a day to using heating pads, but nothing offered lasting relief. "Work was a real challenge," she explains. "My job keeps me very busy, and I was constantly fighting through the pain, just trying to make it through each day." Patty had consulted several doctors, even undergoing an injection for what she thought might be arthritis in her knee. Yet, the aching persisted, and a new, unexpected symptom emerged – her toenails were constantly cold, discolored, and falling off. Even after two years of various treatments, nothing seemed to work.

At Althoff Wellness Clinic PC, we took a different approach. After thorough testing and a detailed review of Patty's medical history, we suspected a possible link between her neuropathy symptoms and gluten sensitivity. We discussed the potential for gluten to trigger inflammation and how it could be impacting her nerve health.

Just six weeks into a personalized REPAIR program that included eliminating gluten from her diet, Patty has experienced a remarkable transformation. "It's almost like night and day," she exclaims. "I can walk up and down the stairs without pain, and I'm finally sleeping through the night!" The relief from pain has also had a positive impact on her energy levels and mood. "I feel so much better overall," she shares. "I can actually participate in life again, and I'm no longer constantly exhausted." Patty's toenails are even showing signs of improvement. "They're not freezing anymore!" she says with a laugh. "And the smaller ones are starting to grow back normally."

While everyone's journey with neuropathy is unique, Patty's story highlights how important it is to explore potential dietary triggers, like gluten, when addressing neuropathy. While more time is needed for full healing, her story offers a powerful example of how eliminating gluten, combined with other elements of the REPAIR program, can lead to significant pain reduction, improved sleep, and a renewed sense of vitality, even in cases where traditional approaches have failed.

Leaky Gut: Beyond Gluten

Gluten is not the only factor that can contribute to a leaky gut. Let's explore other potential causes:

- **Processed Foods and Additives:** Many processed foods contain additives and preservatives that can irritate the gut lining, contributing to increased intestinal permeability.
- **Chronic Stress:** Prolonged stress can weaken the immune system and disrupt the gut barrier function, leading to leaky gut.
- **Medications:** Certain medications, like nonsteroidal anti-inflammatory drugs (NSAIDs) and antibiotics, can damage the gut lining and alter gut flora balance.

- **Infections:** Bacterial, viral, and fungal infections can compromise gut integrity and increase permeability.
- **Environmental Toxins:** Exposure to environmental toxins, such as pesticides and heavy metals, can disrupt gut health and contribute to leaky gut.

Addressing these additional factors is crucial for a comprehensive approach to healing leaky gut and improving neuropathy symptoms.

REPAIR Beyond Gluten: A Multifaceted Approach to Nerve Healing

Removing gluten, if it's a major trigger for you, is a fantastic first step on your journey to reclaiming your health. But let's explore why the REPAIR program is so crucial, even after making this significant dietary change.

Healing is a Journey, Not a Destination: Even with the source of inflammation addressed, existing nerve damage might take time to heal. The therapies in the REPAIR system specifically target stimulating nerve regeneration, boosting blood flow, and calming any lingering inflammation within the nervous system itself.

A Broader View of Inflammation: While incredibly important, gluten may not be the sole culprit when it comes to inflammation. The REPAIR approach takes a comprehensive view, addressing blood sugar imbalances, stress management, and potential nutritional deficiencies – all of which can significantly hamper nerve healing.

Synergy: Building a Superhighway for Healing: Imagine going gluten-free as clearing a path, and the REPAIR therapies as building a superhighway for optimal nerve communication and repair. When combined, they create a force far more potent than either approach could be on its own.

Understanding how gluten and other factors can impact your body is empowering. Regardless of whether it proves to be a major factor in your specific case, this knowledge allows you to make informed choices about your health journey.

By addressing gluten sensitivity (if needed) and utilizing the multifaceted tools of the REPAIR approach, you create the best possible environment for healing and lasting relief from neuropathy. This powerful combination offers a true path to hope and a transformed life.

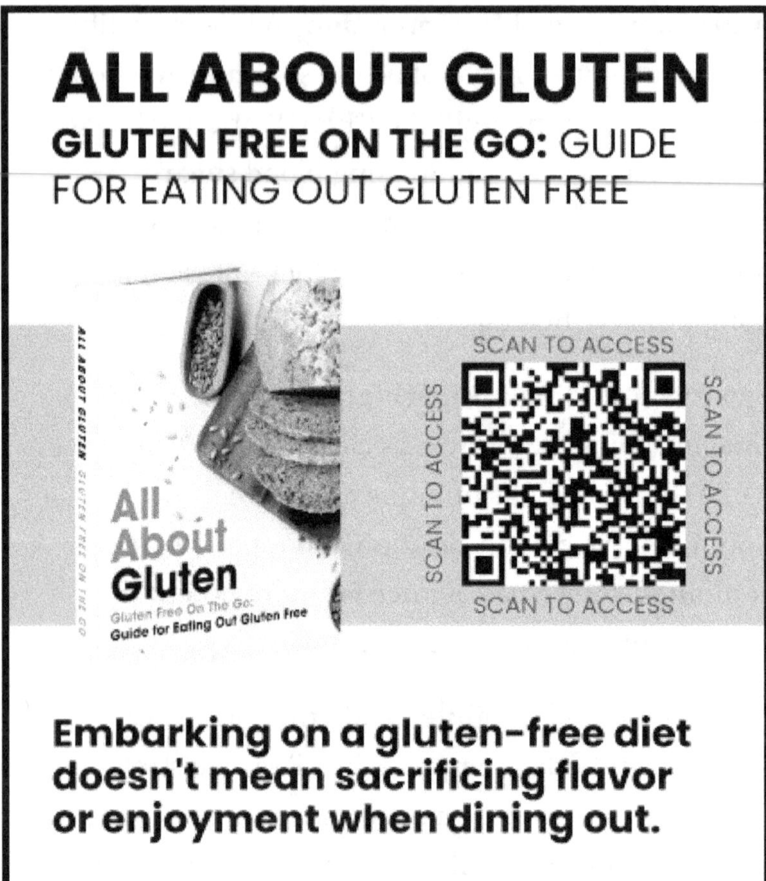

Unlock Your Path to Neuropathy Relief Now: Visit DrJillAlthoff.Com or Call (970) 579-7496 to Speak With Us Today!

Individual results may vary. Please review the disclaimer after the Table of Contents.

11

CIRCULATION AND NEUROPATHY: BOOSTING NERVE REPAIR

Many of our patients tell me they've had their circulation checked. They explain that their primary care physician or neurologist checked the pulse on the top of their foot and behind their ankle. They've often undergone ultrasounds to examine the arteries and veins in their legs. While these methods assess deep arteries and veins, the circulation most affected by neuropathy starts with the surface blood vessels. It's crucial to understand that the health of these smaller, surface vessels plays a significant role in nerve health and can be the first to show signs of poor circulation.

Neuropathy can feel like a complex puzzle with countless pieces. To see the big picture and achieve lasting relief, we need to address all the interconnected factors – inflammation, blood sugar imbalances, nutrient deficiencies, and, crucially, circulation issues. This chapter focuses on improving circulation and exploring several powerful tools that can become significant players in your healing journey. These approaches work within your body's natural healing mechanisms to foster a more favorable environment for nerve repair and reduce symptoms.

Understanding Circulation-Related Neuropathy

Circulation-related peripheral neuropathy is most often experienced by people with diabetes, but anyone with reduced blood circulation is at risk. At Althoff Wellness Clinic, we find that 90% of the patients we see have some sort of circulatory issue. When small blood vessels surrounding the nerves die off, the nerves are deprived of nourishment and eventually also die. These damaged nerves are the source of the pain and tingling experienced by neuropathy sufferers. It is estimated that 60 to 70% of diabetics develop some form of neuropathy. Improving blood flow is, therefore, a critical aspect of managing and healing neuropathy.

Tools to Improve Circulation and Nerve Health

We attack circulatory issues in several different ways within our practice. Some of the most common methods include Low-Level Light Therapy (LLLT), L-

Arginine, and L-Citrulline. However, we also use whole body vibration, extracorporeal shockwave therapy, Class IV laser, pulsed electromagnetic field therapy (pEMF), and NeuroMed. Each of these tools works within your body's natural healing mechanisms to foster a more favorable environment for regeneration and reduce symptoms.

Low-Level Light Therapy: Shining a Light on Neuropathy Relief

Low-Level Light Therapy (LLLT) harnesses the power of light for deep-tissue healing. Imagine it as specialized sunlight, designed to reach and revitalize tissues within your body. LLLT devices use specific wavelengths of red and near-infrared light, unlike heat lamps that emit warmth.

Here's the exciting part: Your cells have tiny power plants called mitochondria, responsible for energy production. These specific light wavelengths get absorbed by the mitochondria, essentially giving them an energy boost. With more energy, your cells can function more efficiently, repair themselves faster, and fight inflammation more effectively.

The science behind LLLT isn't just promising – it's backed by research demonstrating its potential benefits for neuropathy:

- **Reduced Symptoms:** Studies show LLLT can lessen those unpleasant neuropathy sensations (burning, tingling, etc.) while also improving nerve function and balance.
- **Nerve Regeneration:** Lab studies reveal LLLT's ability to promote nerve regrowth after injury, directly benefiting damaged tissues.
- **Improved Blood Flow & Wound Healing:** For those with diabetic neuropathy, LLLT has been shown to improve blood flow and wound healing, crucial aspects of managing this complication.

How Does LLLT Benefit Those with Neuropathy?

- **Taming Inflammation:** Inflammation is a major roadblock to nerve healing. LLLT helps calm inflammation within the tissues, creating a more conducive environment for repair.
- **Boosting Circulation:** Healthy blood flow is crucial for delivering the oxygen and nutrients your nerves need to heal. LLLT stimulates blood vessel formation and improves circulation to damaged areas.
- **Supporting Nerve Regeneration:** LLLT appears to encourage the actual regrowth of damaged nerve fibers. It's not an instant fix, but

it offers hope for reversing the underlying damage of neuropathy.

Putting It into Practice: How to Use LLLT

Now that you understand the potential benefits of Low-Level Light Therapy (LLLT) for neuropathy, you might be wondering how to incorporate it into your routine. Here's a breakdown of the different options available:

- **At-Home Devices:** The good news is that LLLT is accessible! There's a variety of devices available for home use, including pads and handheld units. While convenient, quality matters. Look for devices used in research studies to ensure you're getting an effective product with the proper wavelengths of light.
- **In-Office Treatments:** For those seeking deeper tissue penetration or a more powerful treatment option, some chiropractors and physical therapists offer larger, more high-powered LLLT setups. This can be a good choice for people who prefer a professional setting or have specific areas they want to target. Our office offers Class IV laser treatments, which use high-intensity light beams to penetrate deeply into affected tissues, promoting cellular repair and reducing

inflammation. This non-invasive, drug-free therapy can help improve symptoms of neuropathy by stimulating nerve function, improving circulation, and supporting tissue regeneration.

- **Frequency and Duration:** Consistency is crucial when it comes to LLLT. While results can vary, studies typically show that several treatments per week for several weeks or even months are needed to see significant benefits. Be patient and stick with your treatment plan for optimal results.

Remember, LLLT is often most powerful when used in combination with other approaches in the REPAIR program. These strategies work together to address inflammation, support overall nerve health, and create a comprehensive approach to lasting neuropathy relief.

L-Arginine: A Nitric Oxide Powerhouse for Nerve Repair

Let's talk about L-Arginine, a small but mighty amino acid that plays a crucial role in nerve health. Imagine it as your body's internal construction crew chief, overseeing the critical task of building blood vessel highways to deliver essential supplies.

- **L-Arginine: The Building Block for Nitric Oxide Production**

L-Arginine is an amino acid, one of the building blocks of protein. Your body naturally generates some L-Arginine, and you can also get it from dietary sources like meat, nuts, and dairy products. But here's why it becomes particularly important for neuropathy: L-Arginine is essential for the production of nitric oxide.

Nitric oxide acts like a traffic controller for your blood vessels. When nitric oxide levels are healthy, it signals to blood vessels to relax and widen. This isn't just about blood pressure – it transforms those tiny blood vessels, especially the ones reaching your feet and toes, from congested side streets into multi-lane superhighways.

- **Improved Blood Flow: A Lifeline for Damaged Nerves**

Now picture the delicate nerve fibers in your feet and hands as remote construction sites desperately needing supplies. With poor circulation, oxygen and vital nutrients can barely trickle through, making repairs painfully slow. Good blood flow, boosted by nitric oxide, floods the area with everything needed for healing and rebuilding. It truly acts as a lifeline for those damaged nerves.

- **Beyond Blood Flow: Nitric Oxide's Multifaceted Benefits**

Nitric oxide's benefits for neuropathy extend far beyond just clearing traffic jams within those blood vessel highways. Remember, neuropathy is a double whammy – nerve damage combined with inflammation that hinders repair. Nitric oxide tackles both:

- **Taming Inflammation:** Chronic inflammation is like having constant roadblocks around those damaged nerves. Nitric oxide helps calm this inflammatory response, creating a more conducive environment for healing.
- **The Regeneration Spark:** While research is ongoing, early studies suggest that nitric oxide might directly stimulate the process of nerve regrowth. It's like not only delivering supplies to the construction site (your nerves) but also providing the blueprints for rebuilding.

L-Arginine Supplementation: Considerations and Safety

While you can get L-Arginine from a healthy diet, additional support is often needed when dealing with neuropathy. Here's what you need to consider:

- **Food vs. Supplementation:** L-Arginine-rich foods like meat, poultry, fish, and nuts are great additions to your diet. However, their impact on nitric oxide levels might not be significant enough to promote substantial nerve healing. Supplementation, under the guidance of a healthcare professional, provides a targeted and potentially more impactful dose.

- **Dosage Matters:** There's no magic bullet dosage for L-Arginine with neuropathy. The right amount for you will depend on factors like your overall health and current medications.

- **Safety First:** L-Arginine is generally safe, but it's vital to talk to your doctor before starting any supplements. This is especially important if you take blood pressure medications, as L-Arginine can further lower blood pressure. Your doctor can ensure L-Arginine is the right fit for you and monitor your dosage for optimal benefit and safety.

By incorporating L-Arginine, either through dietary changes or targeted supplementation, you can potentially give your body the tools it needs to improve blood flow, reduce inflammation, and create a more favorable environment for nerve repair – all contributing to lasting neuropathy relief.

L-Citrulline: The Supercharged Ally for Nitric Oxide Production

L-Citrulline can be thought of as L-Arginine's more high-achieving cousin. It's another amino acid found in small amounts in foods like watermelon, but its true power for neuropathy lies in supplementation.

- **Why L-Citrulline? A Sneaky Way to Boost Nitric Oxide**

Just like L-Arginine, L-Citrulline ultimately helps your body produce nitric oxide. But here's the surprising twist: it may be even more effective at doing so! Let's explore why.

Imagine your digestive system as an overzealous security guard. When you take an L-Arginine supplement, a significant portion gets broken down before reaching its intended destination – your bloodstream. This means a lot of that potential benefit is lost.

L-Citrulline, however, is the secret agent of amino acids. It bypasses those gut security guards more easily, leading to better absorption into your bloodstream. Once there, your body efficiently converts it into L-Arginine. In essence, L-Citrulline is a more efficient way to elevate your L-Arginine levels, maximizing the amount that reaches your tissues to promote healing.

L-Citrulline's Multifaceted Benefits for Neuropathy

Since L-Citrulline fuels your body's L-Arginine production, its benefits for neuropathy mirror those of L-Arginine:

- **Enhanced Blood Flow:** The increased nitric oxide tells your blood vessels to relax and widen, transforming those congested side streets leading to your nerves into efficient highways. This improved circulation allows oxygen and vital nutrients to finally reach where they're desperately needed.
- **Reduced Pain:** L-Citrulline offers a double whammy for pain relief. Improved blood flow eases burning or tingling sensations while also addressing the chronic inflammation that often amplifies nerve pain.
- **Potential for Regeneration:** Research suggests L-Citrulline might go beyond just boosting circulation. Early evidence indicates it might even assist in the process of nerve regeneration

itself. Imagine it not just delivering new building materials, but also helping create a more efficient team to rebuild your nerves.

Dosage and Safety: Tailoring Your Approach

As with L-Arginine, L-Citrulline dosages vary based on individual needs. Let's discuss the right amount for you and ensure it doesn't interact with any medications you're currently taking. By incorporating L-Citrulline, you can potentially provide your body with a powerful tool to increase nitric oxide production, improve blood flow, reduce inflammation, and create a more favorable environment for nerve repair – all contributing to lasting neuropathy relief.

Additional Approaches to Improve Circulation

In addition to LLLT, L-Arginine, and L-Citrulline, we also use several other therapies to improve circulation and support nerve health:

- **Whole Body Vibration:** This therapy involves standing on a platform that vibrates at specific frequencies. The vibrations stimulate muscle contractions and improve blood flow, helping to nourish and repair damaged nerves.

- **Extracorporeal Shockwave Therapy:** This non-invasive treatment uses sound waves to stimulate blood vessel formation and improve circulation. It's effective in promoting healing and reducing pain in neuropathy patients.
- **Class IV Laser Therapy:** High-intensity laser beams penetrate deeply into affected tissues, promoting cellular repair, reducing inflammation, and improving circulation. This therapy can significantly enhance nerve function and support tissue regeneration.
- **Pulsed Electromagnetic Field Therapy (pEMF):** pEMF uses electromagnetic fields to stimulate cellular repair and improve blood flow. It helps reduce inflammation and promote healing in damaged nerves.
- **NeuroMed:** This advanced therapy uses electroanalgesia to improve blood flow and reduce pain. It stimulates nerve regeneration and supports overall nerve health.

Patient Journeys: Seeing the Light with RLT and Amino Acids

We've explored the fascinating science behind how L-Arginine and L-Citrulline boost our bodies' natural healing abilities by enhancing blood flow and supporting nerve regeneration. But what does this look like in a person's everyday life? Let's hear from Arlend.

Arlend, an avid golfer, first came to Althoff Wellness Clinic PC with a sense of frustration. Neuropathy had cast a shadow over his favorite pastime. "My feet felt like they were constantly wet and cold," he explains, "hard, almost like blocks of wood. It was really unpleasant." This lack of sensation created a disconcerting sense of imbalance. "I just didn't have that secure footing, especially when walking the course or taking a swing. My balance just wasn't there." Arlend's lack of stability made even simple activities like climbing ladders feel risky, and he was concerned about falling. He longed to reclaim the confidence and joy he once felt on the golf course.

As part of his personalized REPAIR program, Arlend began incorporating Red Light Therapy and targeted amino acid supplementation, including L-Arginine and L-Citrulline. These therapies, along with other vital elements of REPAIR, were carefully chosen to support his nerve health and boost his body's natural healing processes.

Ninety days into the program, Arlend's steps feel lighter, and his smile reflects a newfound hope. "The biggest change I've noticed is my balance," he says, his voice filled with excitement. "Putting on my clothes, swinging the club, even putting—I feel so much more steady and secure now." But the most profound shift for Arlend is the return of sensation to his feet. "I can feel my toes again," he says, a look of wonder in his eyes. "I'm actually feeling the ground beneath my feet, the stones, the little things I didn't even realize I was missing before."

While everyone's journey with neuropathy is unique, Arlend's story is a powerful testament to the potential of these therapies. His journey highlights how red light therapy, L-Arginine, and L-Citrulline can work together to not just improve blood flow and reduce inflammation, but also to reawaken those vital nerve pathways, leading to a significant improvement in both sensation and balance. Arlend's experience is a beacon of hope for anyone seeking to reclaim their mobility and confidently step back into the activities they love.

The REPAIR Program: A Synergistic and Safe Approach to Neuropathy Relief

The REPAIR program centers around the power of synergy – combining tools that amplify each other's effects. This is where the magic happens when we use Low-Level Light Therapy, L-Arginine, L-Citrulline, and other advanced therapies together.

Tackling Neuropathy from Different Angles: A Unified Approach

Imagine each of these elements targeting neuropathy from a unique perspective:

- **Low-Level Light Therapy:** Works at the cellular level, promoting healing by reducing inflammation and encouraging nerve regeneration.
- **L-Arginine & L-Citrulline:** These amino acids work together to optimize blood flow, ensuring crucial oxygen and nutrients reach damaged nerves for repair.
- **Whole Body Vibration, Extracorporeal Shockwave Therapy, Class IV Laser Therapy, pEMF, and NeuroMed:** These therapies further enhance circulation, reduce inflammation, and promote nerve regeneration.

The result? Rather than isolated benefits, these tools work in harmony to create the perfect environment for your nerves to heal. It's a synergistic effect, greater than the sum of its parts.

A Natural Path to Relief

Compared to traditional neuropathy treatments that might focus solely on masking symptoms or carry potential for side effects, the REPAIR program leverages your body's inherent healing mechanisms. This natural approach offers a generally safer and gentler path to lasting relief.

Working with Your Healthcare Team: Individualized Care is Key

While these approaches are natural, it's still crucial to discuss them with your doctor, chiropractor, or other qualified healthcare professional. They can provide personalized dosing recommendations and ensure there are no interactions with any medications you're currently taking. Here at Althoff Wellness Clinic, we prioritize an integrative and individualized approach to conquering neuropathy.

Empowering You to Take Charge of Your Health

We've explored how Low-Level Light Therapy, L-Arginine, L-Citrulline, and other advanced therapies can be powerful allies in your fight against neuropathy. Here's the most important message: these tools work with your body's natural healing potential. They reduce inflammation, improve blood flow, and may even directly support nerve regeneration.

While there's no instant cure, these therapies empower you to take an active role in your health. Instead of just managing symptoms, you're addressing the underlying factors that prevent healing. The REPAIR program provides the optimal environment for your body to do what it does best – repair and rebuild. That's the path to true freedom from the grip of neuropathy.

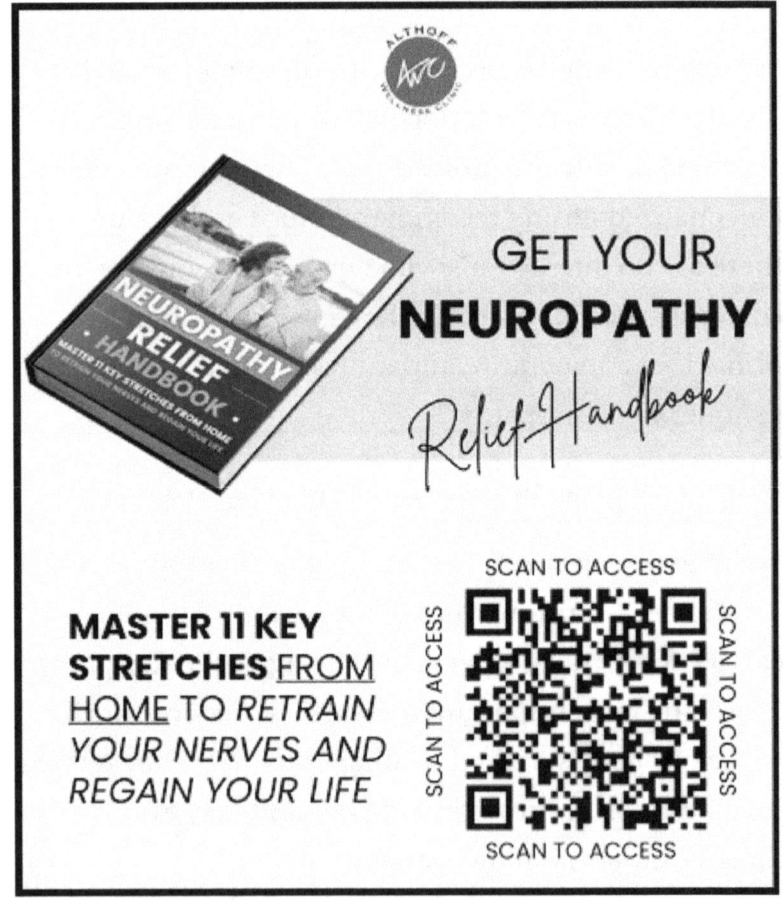

Unlock Your Path to Neuropathy Relief Now: Visit DrJillAlthoff.Com or Call (970) 579-7496 to Speak With Us Today!

157

Individual results may vary. Please review the disclaimer after the Table of Contents.

12

BEYOND ADDICTION: THE HIDDEN COSTS OF OPIOIDS FOR NEUROPATHY

As we explore conquering neuropathy, it's impossible to ignore the other epidemic impacting millions: opioid addiction. Let's be clear – the goal isn't to judge those struggling with addiction but to highlight the very real dangers, especially for people living with the chronic pain of neuropathy.

The statistics are alarming. According to the Centers for Disease Control and Prevention (CDC), more than 1 million people have died since 1999 from a drug overdose, and more than 75% of drug overdose deaths involved opioids. It's a vicious cycle – someone in constant agony seeks relief through medication, often unaware of the potential consequences.

Neuropathy creates a perfect storm for opioid vulnerability. The unrelenting burning, tingling, or electric shock sensations can push even the most resilient person to a breaking point. In those moments of desperation, powerful pain medications can appear to be the only answer.

While there may be rare cases where very short-term opioid use is necessary under strict medical supervision, it's crucial to understand the risks involved. What might initially feel like a lifesaver can quickly morph into a dangerous trap.

Opioids for Neuropathy: Masking Pain, Not Repairing Damage

Opioids can be a double-edged sword for neuropathy. While they may offer a tempting illusion of relief, they don't address the root cause of the problem. Let's delve into why they might not be the most effective solution.

Pain Masking, Not Healing: Opioids work by essentially blocking pain signals before they reach your brain. Imagine them as cutting the wires to a fire alarm. The fire itself continues to burn, but the warning siren is silenced. You might feel relief, but the underlying nerve damage causing those neuropathy symptoms remains unaddressed.

The Tolerance Trap: Our bodies are remarkably adaptable. With prolonged use, your body builds tolerance to opioids, meaning the same dose no longer provides the same level of pain relief. This creates a dangerous cycle. In the quest to recapture that initial numbing effect, people often escalate their opioid use, increasing dosage or frequency. The focus shifts from managing pain to simply avoiding withdrawal symptoms.

The Risk-Reward Imbalance: Long-term opioid use carries a significant risk of addiction, dependence, and even overdose. Considering they don't address the underlying cause of neuropathy, the potential downsides outweigh the limited benefits.

There are far more effective and sustainable ways to manage neuropathy pain. The REPAIR neuropathy program offers a comprehensive approach that can address the root cause of your neuropathy and provide lasting relief.

The Ripple Effects of Opioids: Beyond the Risk of Addiction

Opioids for neuropathy come with a hidden price tag, extending far beyond the well-known risk of addiction. Even when taken as prescribed, side effects can significantly impact your quality of life and even worsen neuropathy itself.

The Physical Burden

- **Constipation:** Severe constipation isn't just uncomfortable – it can have cascading effects. Straining can aggravate existing health issues, while backed-up toxins worsen inflammation, a major roadblock to healing neuropathy.
- **Brain Fog:** Opioids can cause a fuzzy, disoriented feeling that goes beyond mere inconvenience. When you're already dealing with the cognitive challenges of neuropathy, this added mental fog makes daily tasks and social interactions incredibly difficult.
- **Hormonal Havoc:** Opioids disrupt your delicate hormonal balance, manifesting in sleep disturbances (making neuropathy pain harder to manage), low mood and irritability, and even metabolic changes affecting weight and energy levels. This overall decline in well-being makes fighting neuropathy even more uphill.

Opioids and Worsening Neuropathy: A Catch-22

Emerging research reveals a concerning link between opioids and long-term nerve damage – a major reason why seeking alternative pain management methods for neuropathy is vital. Here's why.

Potential Mechanisms of Opioid-Induced Nerve Damage:

- **Increased Inflammation and Oxidative Stress:** Opioids may exacerbate inflammation and oxidative stress, further harming already compromised nerves.
- **Direct Nerve Damage:** There's a possibility opioids might directly damage sensory receptors within the nerves themselves.
- **Delayed Intervention:** By suppressing pain signals, opioids might prevent you from seeking other therapies that could actually address the root cause of neuropathy.

A Downward Spiral: The Opioid Trap

Here's a glimpse into the vicious cycle opioids can create, particularly for neuropathy patients:

- **Desperate Relief:** You begin taking opioids for pain relief, and initially, they seem effective.

- **Tolerance & The Illusion of Control:** Over time, your body develops tolerance, and the pain starts to creep back. Thinking "more is better," you increase the dose (sometimes without your doctor's knowledge). This offers temporary relief but unknowingly worsens underlying neuropathy.
- **Repeat and Escalate:** The cycle repeats. More pain necessitates a higher dose, further escalating the problem.

Because opioids mask pain perception, it feels like they're solving the issue. However, the underlying damage continues, making you believe you need the medication even more. The drug slowly transforms from a pain management tool to the very source of your pain.

Breaking free from this cycle is incredibly challenging due to the physical dependence. This is why it's crucial to address neuropathy pain at its source and explore safer, more effective alternatives before the risk of addiction takes hold.

Escaping the Opioid Cycle: Hope and Practical Steps

Breaking free from opioid dependence is undeniably challenging, but it's a journey filled with hope. This message is crucial – you can reclaim your life from pain and medication dependence. There's no shame in seeking help; opioid addiction can happen to anyone facing unrelenting pain. The first step towards a brighter future is acknowledging you need support, and there are excellent resources available.

Safe Tapering: A Must for Success

Going "cold turkey" is incredibly dangerous. Abruptly stopping opioids triggers severe withdrawal symptoms like:

- Intense muscle aches and flu-like symptoms
- Crippling anxiety, restlessness, and insomnia
- Digestive issues (nausea, diarrhea, vomiting)
- Fluctuations in blood pressure and heart rate

The severity varies, but the experience is undeniably awful. This is why attempting to quit without medical guidance is so risky. It often leads to relapse simply to find relief, even with the strongest desire to break free.

An addiction medicine specialist can create a personalized, slow-tapering plan considering your individual dose and usage history. This significantly reduces withdrawal symptoms, making them more manageable. While still difficult, the process becomes more tolerable, increasing your chances of success.

The REPAIR Neuropathy Program: A Sustainable Solution

The key to lasting freedom lies in addressing the root cause of your pain – the neuropathy itself. Instead of simply numbing symptoms, the REPAIR program focuses on healing the damaged nerves. As the pain naturally lessens and function improves, your reliance on medication decreases organically. This offers a sustainable path forward, not just a temporary solution.

The REPAIR program provides you with a comprehensive approach to address the underlying causes of neuropathy and promote lasting relief. We'll explore various tools and strategies to empower you to manage your pain naturally and effectively, reducing your dependence on opioids and reclaiming your quality of life.

Breaking the Chains: Preventing Opioid Dependence

Let's shift gears and focus on preventing this devastating cycle from ever taking hold. The key lies in proactive neuropathy management and open communication with your healthcare team.

The longer neuropathy pain goes unaddressed, the greater the risk of turning to opioids in desperation. Seeking REPAIR program-like care as soon as possible is vital. When pain is effectively managed from the outset, the temptation of risky quick fixes like opioids significantly diminishes.

Open Communication is Key

Be upfront with your doctor about the severity of your neuropathy pain, even if you fear judgment. Don't downplay your suffering! Honest communication allows us to explore safer alternatives early on – targeted therapies, specific exercises, or non-opioid pain management strategies tailored to your unique needs.

Battling Addiction: Compassion and Hope

Battling opioid addiction takes immense courage, and the journey is far from easy. It's important to offer compassion towards those struggling and remind them that addiction doesn't define them – it can be overcome.

There's a different path available, one that leads to true healing, not just masked pain. Whether you're concerned about yourself or a loved one, the REPAIR program offers a powerful alternative.

REPAIR: Healing Beyond the Physical

True healing doesn't just address the physical symptoms of neuropathy – it protects your overall well-being and empowers you to reclaim control over your life. The REPAIR program offers a comprehensive approach that can address the root cause of your neuropathy and promote lasting relief, naturally and effectively.

Let's explore ways to manage your pain without resorting to opioids and pave the way for a brighter, healthier future.

Bud's Story: Finding Relief and Hope Beyond Medication

Bud, a cancer survivor, first came to Althoff Wellness Clinic PC after enduring years of relentless neuropathy pain following chemotherapy. "The pain in my feet was so bad, especially at night," Bud recalls, his voice tinged with the memory of sleepless nights. "It kept me awake constantly. I couldn't even relax in a warm bath because the pain was so intense."

Bud was determined to avoid strong pain medications, having witnessed their devastating side effects firsthand. "Pain meds make me terribly sick," he shares. "So I didn't take anything for the pain." But the unrelenting discomfort took a toll, not just physically but also emotionally. "The lack of sleep, the constant pain—it affected me deeply," Bud confides. "I was struggling with depression and had to rely on antidepressants just to cope."

Like many others, Bud had consulted multiple doctors who offered little hope for relief. "They all said the same thing—there's nothing that can fix neuropathy, you just have to learn to live with it," Bud recounts, his voice heavy with the weight of that prognosis.

However, Bud refused to accept a life defined by pain and medication dependence. When he heard about Althoff Wellness Clinic PC and the REPAIR program, he felt a flicker of hope. "I wanted to believe it could help," he says, "but honestly, after all those other doctors, I wasn't sure." Despite his skepticism, Bud chose to embrace the opportunity for a different approach.

Today, Bud's story is one of resilience and renewed hope. "The REPAIR program has made a huge difference," he shares, his face radiant. "The pain is so much less now. It doesn't bother me like it used to, and I can finally sleep through the night!" The relief from pain has had a ripple effect on Bud's overall well-being. "I've become more active, and I'm off all the antidepressants now!" he exclaims. "I feel like I have my life back. I feel like myself again."

Individual results may vary. However, Bud's journey highlights that hope and healing are possible without resorting to the risky path of opioids. His story demonstrates that by addressing the root causes of neuropathy and embracing a holistic approach to pain management, you can break free from the cycle of suffering and rediscover a life filled with possibility.

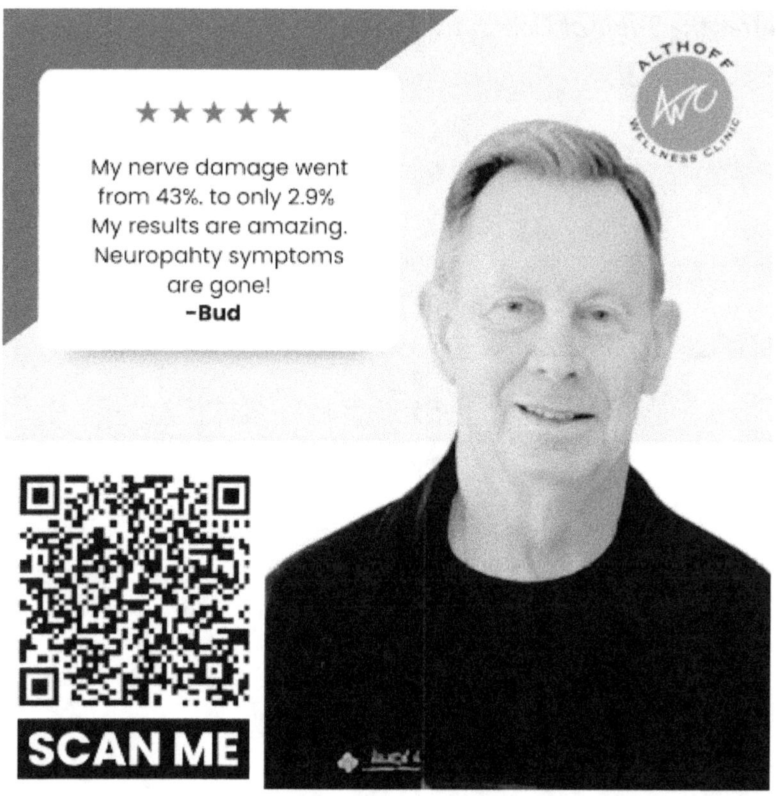

Unlock Your Path to Neuropathy Relief Now: Visit DrJillAlthoff.Com or Call (970) 579-7496 to Speak With Us Today!

Individual results may vary. Please review the disclaimer after the Table of Contents.

13

YOUR INVITATION TO BLOOM: EMBRACING THE REPAIR JOURNEY

There's a particular kind of magic that happens when a patient rediscovers their confidence. It's a quiet victory, a subtle shift in their gaze, a newfound lightness in their step. I saw this transformation firsthand with Gloria. When she first came to Althoff Wellness Clinic PC, her eyes held a familiar blend of fear and resignation. Neuropathy had stolen her sense of security, making her hesitant even to walk across the room. But 71 days into the REPAIR program, I witnessed something remarkable. Gloria walked into my office, not with tentative steps but with a purposeful stride. Her face, once etched with worry, now radiated a quiet joy. "I didn't realize how unsteady I'd become until I felt that confidence come back," she confessed, tears welling up in her eyes. It was a profound moment, a testament to the power of reclaiming not just physical function but also the very essence of self-belief.

It's important to remember that every patient's journey is unique. However, Gloria's story reminds us that a holistic approach can bring about a profound transformation, not just in physical function but also in a person's sense of self-worth and ability to embrace life fully.

We stand at the precipice of a transformative adventure, dear reader. This is not just the end of a book; it's the beginning of a vibrant tapestry you weave with your own hands, a journey towards reclaiming your well-being with the REPAIR neuropathy program as your guide.

You've delved into the depths of neuropathy, explored the power of REPAIR principles, and glimpsed the potential for a future overflowing with vibrant nerve health. Now, it's time to make a decisive commitment, to step boldly onto the path towards a life unburdened by discomfort, a life brimming with possibility.

Embrace the REPAIR Journey, and:

Reimagine Your Future: Let go of the limitations imposed by neuropathy and envision a future where you move freely, feel deeply, and thrive with unbridled vitality. The possibilities are endless, waiting to be painted onto your canvas of well-being.

Unleash Your Inner Healer: REPAIR equips you with the knowledge and tools to become the architect of your own recovery. You'll learn to nourish your nerves, cultivate mindful movement, and build a sustainable routine that fuels your journey for years to come.

Experience the Power of Community: You're not alone on this path. The REPAIR community offers unwavering support, shared wisdom, and a sense of belonging. Together, we'll lift each other up and celebrate every victory, big or small.

Ready to Take the First Step?

Claim Your Private 1-on-1 Consultation: Discover how a holistic approach can help manage your neuropathy pain without relying on harmful medications or procedures.

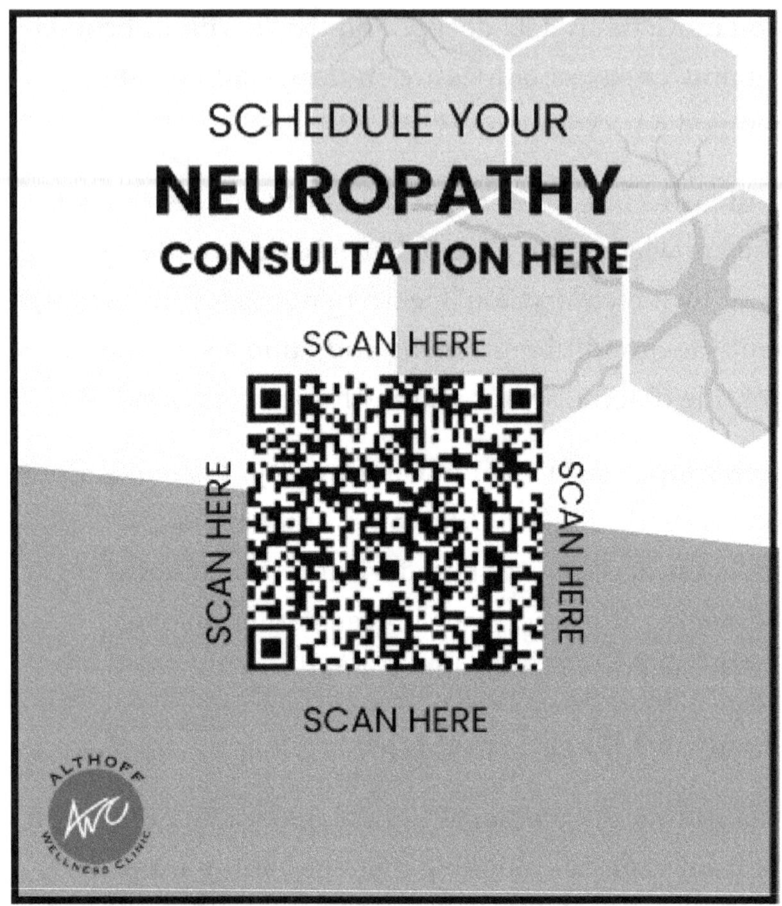

Not anywhere near Windsor, CO, or Cheyenne, WY?
Then watch our free "3 Secrets to Reversing
Neuropathy" masterclass by scanning the code below.

Remember, the path to well-being is paved with action. Step onto it with courage, embrace the REPAIR journey with open arms, and watch your life blossom with newfound joy, freedom, and vibrant nerve health.

The time to reclaim your well-being is now. Let's bloom together, one mindful step, one joyful movement, and one transformative choice at a time.

I look forward to welcoming you to the REPAIR program and witnessing your remarkable journey unfold!